BACH
FLOWER
MASSAGE

BACH
FLOWER
MASSAGE

DANIELE LO RITO, M.D.
Translated from the Italian by Tami Calliope

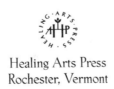

Healing Arts Press
Rochester, Vermont

Healing Arts Press
One Park Street
Rochester, Vermont 05767
www.gotoit.com

First English language edition published by Healing Arts Press 1997

Originally published in Italian under the title Il Massagio con i fiori di Bach by Xenia
Edizioni 1995

Copyright © 1995, 1997 Xenia Edizioni, Via dell'Annunciata 31, Milano, Italy
Translation copyright © 1997 by Inner Traditions International

*Note to the reader: This book is intended as an informational guide. The remedies, approaches, and
techniques described herein are meant to supplement, and not to be a substitute for, professional
medical care or treatment. They should not be used to treat a serious ailment without prior consultation
with a qualified health-care professional.*

Library of Congress Cataloging-in-Publication Data

Lo Rito, Daniele.
    [Massagio con i fiori di Bach.   English]
    Bach flower massage / Daniele Lo Rito ; translated from the Italian by Tami
Calliope.
        p.   cm.
    Includes bibliographical references.
    ISBN 0-89281-736-4 (alk. paper)
    1. Flowers—Therapeutic use. 2. Massage. 3. Bach, Edward, 1886–1936.
I. Title.
RX615.F55L613   1997   97-26253
615'.321—dc21   CIP

Printed and bound in the United States

10 9 8 7 6 5 4 3 2 1

Text design and layout by Kristin Camp
This book was typeset in Garamond with Phaistos as the display typeface

Healing Arts Press is a division of Inner Traditions International

Distributed to the book trade in Canada by Publishers Group West (PGW), Toronto, Ontario
Distributed to the health food trade in Canada by Alive Books, Toronto and Vancouver
Distributed to the book trade in the United Kingdom by Deep Books, London
Distributed to the book trade in Australia by Millennium Books, Newtown, N.S.W.
Distributed to the book trade in New Zealand by Tandem Press, Auckland
Distributed to the book trade in South Africa by Alternative Books, Ferndale

I dedicate this book
to that angel
named Antonella
who instills in me
her energies,
her wisdom,
and the eternal love of Eve
so that I may find myself once more
united with Him.

—Daniele

CONTENTS

ACKNOWLEDGMENTS

I thank all the friends who have helped me with the drafting of this text, and send them an eternal sigh of love.

An acknowledgment of light to those invisible beings who animate nature and and help humankind to walk on the path of Harmony. To these Angels I send an eternal impulse of joy, so happy am I to hear and see them.

Thank you all for the love you have given me, for the time you've put into the work, and for the energies you have so generously shared.

INTRODUCTION

The creative impulse behind this book was born many years ago when I became interested for a prolonged period of time in the studies of Doctor Calligaris concerning the discovery of the psyche's effect on the skin and vice versa. These studies were explorations of the principle which proposed that, by stimulating certain areas of the skin, it is possible to evoke specific feelings—and that there are feelings specific to every area of the skin. Thus love, compassion, hatred, or anger could each sensitize in some way its own unique and reflexive skin zones.

Some years later, following my own studies in iridology and *cronorischio*—my term for the record of past traumas found on the front part of the iris—I once again stumbled upon the idea that the skin might be a kind of mnemonic storage system. By analysis of the rim of the corona, situated at the level of the iris, it is possible to backtrack to the age at which the individual suffered physical and psychic trauma, either in life or while in the womb. The next step was to locate on a cutaneous level the same information encountered in the iris and to verify the sensitivity of the individual traumatized zones. My clinical experiences confirmed this working hypothesis on the interconnection between traumatic event and skin, trauma and iris. Mindful of Doctor Calligaris's research, I began to stimulate the skin zones linked to the cronorischio and was able to verify, to my own amazement, that this reawakened the feelings experienced at the time of original trauma.

During this time I was also devoting myself to Bach flower therapy and the study of therapeutic flowers from California, Alaska, and

Australia. I began to apply these floral essences to certain areas of the skin and observed that they not only relieved local disturbances—such as paresthesia, muscular contractions, and rigidity—but also acted on the emotional and psychic planes. Subsequent study of the exogenous medicine of Doctor Mandel and of the contributions of Dietmar Krämer enriched the research I had been conducting. I am deeply grateful to these authors, who by their studies have contributed so much to our holistic understanding of this marvelous being named man. In this text, therefore, I have reassembled the invaluable discoveries of these scholars, confirmed by my experience, in hopes of providing the reader with a diagnostic and therapeutic tool of extreme practicality and efficacy.

As Rudolf Steiner said, the therapy of the future will work through stimulation of the skin and applications of substances absorbed by the epithelium.

I will never cease to be astonished by the unexpected wonders I see in the course of my work. By analysis of active and silent cutaneous zones, it is possible to isolate one or more flower essence correspondent to the psychic and emotional picture. It is surprising to observe the physical and emotional changes that occur after even a short and very light stimulation of the skin; often the application of the flower essence alone will lessen the stomachache, loosen the cramped muscle, or cause patients to declare that the anxiety or internal tremor from which they were suffering is gone, yet I had only grazed the skin or dabbed it with a flower-essence cream. We may infer from this that the skin acts as an experiential reflection of states of inner imbalance, as well as of cosmic and archetypal influences beyond the reach of the conscious-yet-perceptible through this sensual apparatus. Skin: the boundary between being and nonbeing, between placement in space and the infinite, between personal and collective.

THE SKIN ZONES: A TOPOGRAPHY OF THE EMOTIONS

The skin of the human body presents an almost magical mirror, invisible to ordinary sight, in which the whole inner world of a person is reflected. Cutaneous tissue is the repository of archetypal memory, from which the cerebral cortex obtains its bits of information, filing them away when it deems them no longer useful. Yet a basic psychocutaneous reflection exists, by which feelings, thoughts, and emotions sensitize a certain area of the skin, sometimes to the point of hypersensitivity. By an analysis of skin zones, therefore, we can identify the emotions that have disturbed the client that day or in preceding days, and by the stimulation of the pertinent skin zones we can actually evoke the correspondent emotion.

It follows that the brain is only an indirect producer of thought, in that it simply elaborates on information originating in the outer world, always processed, however, through a whole series of memories inscribed in the genetic code.

The skin must be seen as an organ of multiple functions and purposes. In fact it is in the skin that the neurological organs delegated to sensitivity are encountered, along with the meridians of acupuncture, the points outside meridians, and the reflexive skin zones of Calligaris, Mandel, or Krämer—and those are the few areas we know something about.

The skin represents the visible confines of the physical body, where information, vibration, and colors take on corporality. It is the sensitive paper on which the various etheric bodies and other subtle bodies imprint themselves, translating messages from the invisible world to the world of appearance.

Skin zones are divided into *active areas* and *silent areas:*

- **Active areas** are corporal zones that clearly demonstrate the necessity for healing through symptoms like numbness or tingling, itching, hypersensitivity, skin eruptions, flushing, changing color, aches and pains, or inelasticity. These areas, by way of cutaneous topography, indicate directly which flower we should use and whether we should use it locally or orally.
- **Silent areas** are cutaneous zones in which no evident signs of paresthetic or chromatic change are manifested. Either there is an alteration of the auric field, which has not yet translated itself into a physical disturbance, or else the central site remains quiet and the disturbance breaks out in another skin zone

corresponding to the same flower essence. Then again, there are situations in which the disturbance has been cured by oral means, yet remains alive as a memory at the cutaneous level.

It is advisable to work on all the areas affected by the same flower essence, stimulating them within an area about three-eighths of an inch in diameter, one at a time, starting with the most active and ending with the least active. Remember to monitor all the affected skin zones, as there is always the potential for displacement of activity from one zone to another.

INDICATIONS, CONTRAINDICATIONS, AND PROPHYLAXIS

Before beginning an evocative cutaneous therapy, we must know the cause of the disturbance manifesting on the surface to ascertain that it is not a masked form of acute or chronic inflammation, potentially life-threatening to the individual in question. An accurate diagnosis and a detailed case history are the necessary tools that permit us to work serenely and efficiently.

The physical disturbances that may be treated in this way are:

- muscular aching and pain after strain
- contractions of the vertebral and paravertebral musculature
- headaches due to muscular tension or stress
- slight burns, wounds, and abrasions
- acne and blackheads
- cutaneous consequences of violent and sudden emotions (anger, rage, hatred, etc.)
- light cases of rhinitis (an inflammation of the mucous membranes of the nose)
- continual fatigue
- muscle cramps
- itching or hyperaesthesia of the skin
- post-herpetic aching and pain

- combined with focused and specific medical therapies
- cutaneous scars, as sites of secondary disturbance (theory of secondaries).

This treatment is *contraindicated* in cases of:

- suppurations of the skin
- serious or extensive burns
- exposed fractures
- skin tumors (melanoma, spinocellular carcinoma, etc.)
- tumorous abscesses.

Evocative cutaneous treatment can be used as preventive therapy in cases involving:

- intense emotional changes, which show at first analysis a disturbance in the aura and secondarily a physical damage (by understanding the emotion that provoked the disturbance, we can locate the correspondent skin zones and treat them with the appropriate flower essence for a prolonged period of time);
- profound and painful spiritual conflict, in the initial phase;
- post-traumatic therapy.

WAYS TO USE THE ESSENCES AND THERAPEUTIC REACTIONS

The flower essences can be used in conjunction with:

- medical therapies involving chemical, homeopathic, or natural means
- oral flower-essence therapy
- psychotherapeutic techniques
- acupuncture
- color therapy
- different skin zones
- different flower essences.

But they may also be used by themselves, in the form of:

Creams—by using a cream with a natural base (jojoba, for instance) containing specific flower essences. You can buy these already prepared and mixed. You can stimulate the skin before applying the cream or after rubbing it in. Apply once a day, twice in more complicated cases.

Bandages—by placing a hypoallergenic bandage spread with flower-essence cream on the correspondent zone, and leaving it in place for 12 to 24 hours.

Compresses—by putting two drops or more of the flower essence(s) in a quarter of a glass of water. Soak a cloth in the water and apply for 10 minutes to the predetermined skin zone, at least once a day.

To avoid violent therapeutic reaction it is advisable not to massage the skin zone directly with the flower essences right away in serious or more complicated cases. It is better to begin with compresses or daily application of the cream for a week, working up to an eventual massage.

The patient him- or herself should massage the pertinent skin zone. If this is not possible, the therapist who gives the massage must be capable of very swiftly absorbing and discarding the negative vibrations of his subject. In fact, direct transferences of physical or emotional symptoms from the patient to the therapist do occur.

Pay very close attention to the skin zones and to the instructions regarding light or strong massage. *Never disregard* these instructions as doing so may provoke violent and undesirable reactions, and result in arousing the opposite of the emotion you wished to evoke. When using flower essences, keep in mind the following:

- Pure flower essences are extremely strong, so it is advisable to dilute them.
- When you have identified a transference of symptoms from one skin zone to another, the second zone should be treated until healing occurs.

- Sometimes healing occurs through a dream, even a troubled and tortured one.
- Stimulation must be applied very lightly to evoke the feeling that corresponds to the skin zone, and energetically whenever you want to evoke the opposite emotion (for example, by stimulating the zone of concord lightly I evoke concord; by stimulating it energetically I evoke discord). Thus in the same zone we have a double possibility: to evoke the feeling or its opposite.

AGE AS REPRESENTED ON THE CUTANEOUS LEVEL

An intense emotion, tied to a trauma suffered years before, may remain alive and apparently insurmountable in some individuals. But by way of flower essences we can harmonize and bring into balance this emotion, a record of which is still conserved in the skin zone and linked with the client's age at the time of trauma. At this point we can turn to an accurate case history or to iridology, by way of an analysis of the cronorischio.

In the eye, on the rim of the corona, we can "read" the circle of life that begins at birth to form on the front part of the iris and, moving around the circumference counterclockwise, completes a quarter of a circle every fifteen years.

It is possible to carry out this same procedure on the skin, at various levels of localization. Once the year of the stressful event has been precisely determined, the corresponding area, which will be hyperaesthetic or painful to the touch, can be examined. Once identified, it can be evaluated according to one of several methods:

- by very, very lightly grazing the skin with a feather;
- by application of the flower essence corresponding to the emotion or psychic state evoked in the individual by the past trauma;
- by stimulation of the skin combined with application of the flower essence, mixed into cream or diluted;
- by application of the floral cream on a bandage, to be left in place.

The skin must be massaged for about ten minutes or more in a silent environment, with the patient's eyes closed so that she may conjure up visually as well as emotionally those feelings bound to the memories in her skin. We must all free ourselves of the baggage of our emotional memories, which ties us to the past and keeps us from living freely in the present.

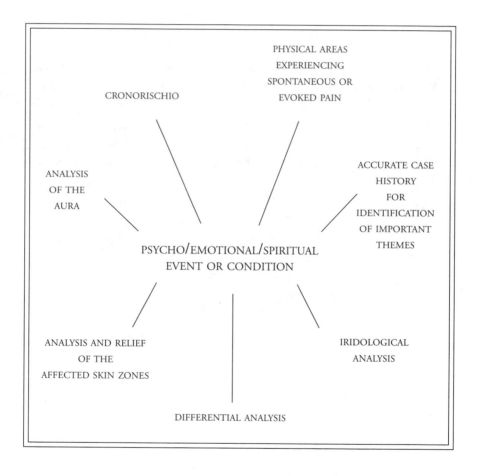

FIGURE 1. DIAGRAM OF DIAGNOSIS

The application of the flower essence must be repeated many times over a month or more of therapy, leaving time for reaction and restoration of balance between one application and another. In more serious and complicated cases it is well to entrust the client to the care of a therapist for the eventual management of unforeseeable reactions and for counseling and treatment.

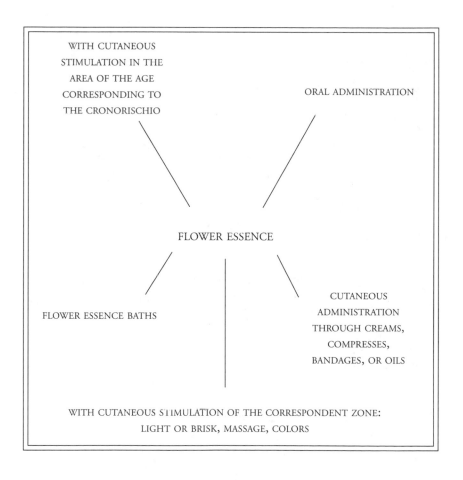

WITH CUTANEOUS STIMULATION IN THE AREA OF THE AGE CORRESPONDING TO THE CRONORISCHIO

ORAL ADMINISTRATION

FLOWER ESSENCE

FLOWER ESSENCE BATHS

CUTANEOUS ADMINISTRATION THROUGH CREAMS, COMPRESSES, BANDAGES, OR OILS

WITH CUTANEOUS STIMULATION OF THE CORRESPONDENT ZONE: LIGHT OR BRISK, MASSAGE, COLORS

FIGURE 2. DIAGRAM OF THERAPY

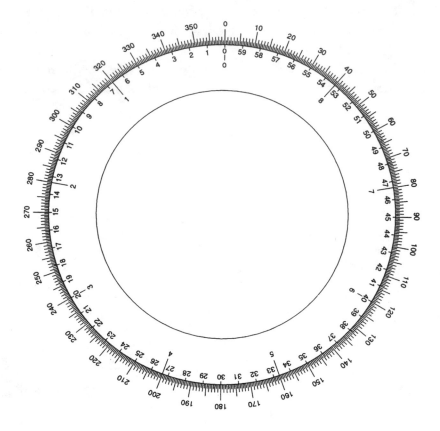

FIGURE 3. GRAPH OF THE IRIDOLOGICAL CRONORISCHIO
PROJECTED ONTO THE CUTANEOUS LEVEL

Reproduced here are some geometric figures that can be helpful in evocative cutaneous therapy. They must be used in sequence, starting from the point corresponding to the traumatic event. These diagrams must be used one at a time and with caution, as there are many possible ways to identify and treat cronorischio through the use of geometric figures. I describe only the simplest of them here, by means of which we will examine a trauma suffered at the age of ten (see Figures 4, 5, 6, and 7).

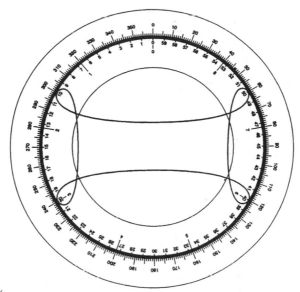

FIGURE 4

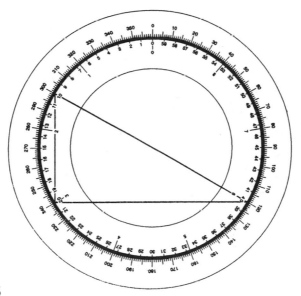

FIGURE 5

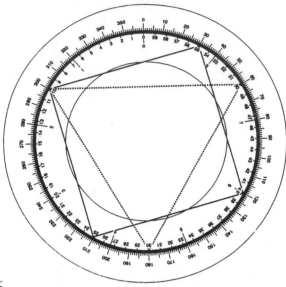

FIGURE 6

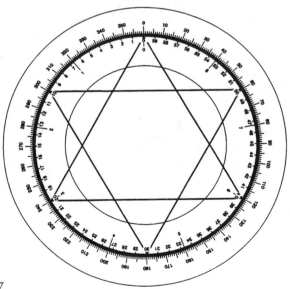

FIGURE 7

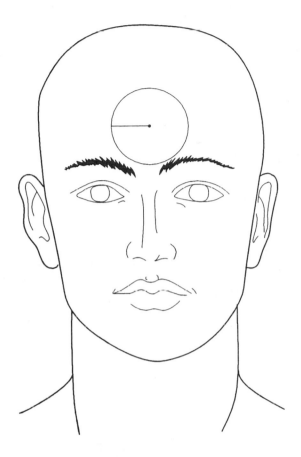

FIGURE 8

First let me describe, in brief, the principal *anterior skin zones* in which we most frequently encounter representations of the patient's age by means of a circular diagram. The topographic skin zones in which we may read the patient's age (at the time of trauma) are many and have a different spatial relationship to the anterior–posterior, horizontal–vertical–oblique, and high–low planes, to mention a few.

Frontal zone: The circle (Figure 8) has its center in the middle of the forehead with a spoke that touches the vertical line passing through the center of the pupil. This is the central circle of the three concentric circles evidenced on the forehead; the spokes of the other two reach respectively to the vertical line passing through the internal and external canthus of the eye.

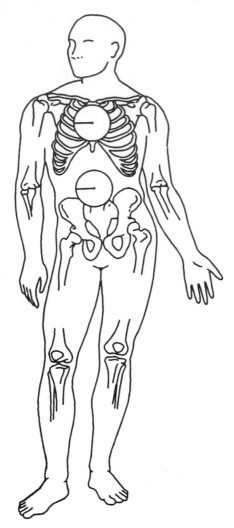

FIGURE 9

Conception and birth are located at the highest point of the circle, that is, at zero degrees, moving counterclockwise to the lowest point of the circle, representing thirty years of age. For traumatic prenatal events, the circle is divided into nine months, so that one month occupies forty degrees of circumference.

Anterior thoracic zone: The circle (Figure 9) has its center at the level of the CV18 point of acupuncture, equivalent to half the length of the sternum, with a spoke touching the mammillary line. This circle lies between the circle whose spoke passes through the parasternal line and the circle whose spoke passes through the anterior axilla. The topographic representation follows the same general principle, in that conception and birth are located in the upper part and subsequent years are counted in a counterclockwise fashion.

Abdominal zone: The circle (Figure 9) has its center at the level of the umbilicus with a spoke that touches the lower extension of the mammillary line. This circle lies between the circle whose spoke touches the extension of the parasternal line and the circle of the anterior axillary line. The topographic arrangement is the same.

THE
THIRTY-EIGHT
BACH FLOWER
ESSENCES

1
Agrimony
Agrimonia eupatoria

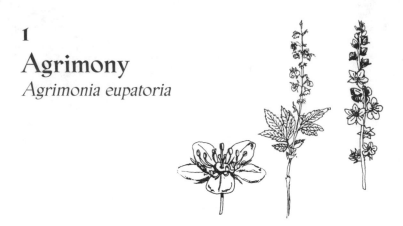

Family: Rosaceae

Habitat: Widespread throughout North America and northern Europe except in arctic regions. Agrimony grows in clayey soils, near ditches, along roadsides, and in pastures at elevations up to 3,500 feet.

Description: Perennial herbaceous plant, up to 28 inches high, with a simple erect, velvety, cylindrical stem. The leaves are pinnately compound, formed from 5 to 9 alternate, serrated leaflets to 5 to 10 smaller leaflets with grayish undersides and stipules. The flowers, composed of 5 petals, 10 to 20 stamens, 2 styles, and a hook-shaped calyx, are numerous, small, and yellow, borne in long terminal spikes. Agrimony flowers from June through September.

Qualities:

- Inner peace
- Capacity for confrontation
- Joy, not only in social behavior
- Integration of difficulties
- Understanding of and ability to work with emotional pain
- Recognition of the shadow self
- Openness to that which is concealed

Indicated for: those who have difficulty integrating their experiences and who resist making contact with the inner and most profound parts of themselves. Such people find it a hardship to express themselves, almost as if they were without a common language with which to communicate. They may live in a condition of conflict and interior suffering because their souls have not managed to amalgamate the two polarities. Restless and tormented, in spiritual pain, they are unable to give expression to their inner sufferings. Since Agrimony individuals seldom seek help or share confidences, not even their closest friends can fully understand the ebb and flow of their thoughts. They become perfect actors, archetypes of the clown who at any cost must make himself and others merry; they always appear to be happy, cordial, and lighthearted, ready to joke around even when they are physically ill. They throw themselves headlong into every activity, every invitation to party; and while they are wonderful company, they are afraid to be by themselves. They are forever seeking acceptance and long to be welcomed. At some point in their lives they may seek, albeit rarely, refuge in stimulants such as alcohol and "uppers," in order to maintain a social role constructed over the years. They may also suffer from longstanding and unresolved problems, held hidden in the unconscious.

I am at peace and content within myself.
Harmony reigns in my inner world.

Skin Zones of Agrimony

A   Nasal zone: extends from the midpoint of the eyebrows down the center of the nose to its tip and around its base, covering the whole left side of the nose.
Massage: *light.*

B Abdominal zone: extends in an oval whose center is located exactly halfway between the xiphoid process and the navel.
Massage: *light*.

C Wrist zone: extends in an oval on the lefthand and righthand wrists, over the pulse.
Massage: *light*.

D Right thoracic zone: extends in a ½-inch-large area on the median axillary line, 3 finger widths under the fold of the armpit.
Massage: *light*.

E Left pelvic zone: a 1⅛-inch-high rectangle whose horizontal bottom line lies over the pubic bone, starting at the linea alba and extending leftward for 4 inches.
Massage: *light*.

F Lumbosacral zone: extends about 1½ inches to the right and left of the line of the tailbone.
Massage: *light*.

G Zone at the back of the upper right thigh: extends along the median line of the thigh from the fold of the buttock to the popliteal.
Massage: *light*.

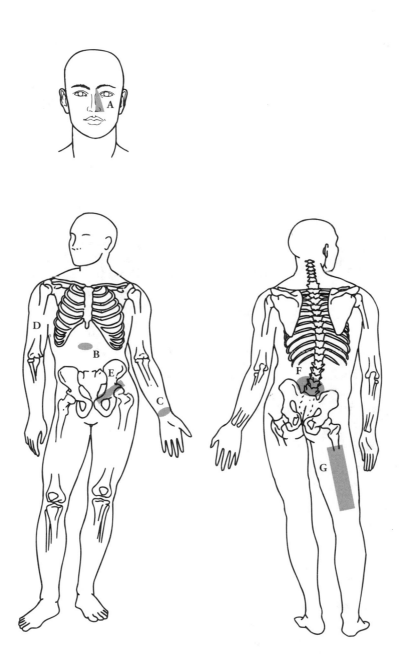

AGRIMONY

2
Aspen
Populus tremula (Quaking Aspen)

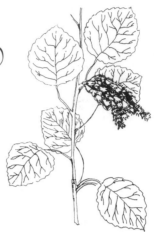

Family: Salicaceae

Habitat: Present in North America, Europe, Asia, and Africa, where it grows in the humid forests of plains, hills, and mountains up to 5,000 or 6 ,000 feet. It is often associated with chestnut, beech, maple, and oak. A light-loving plant, it does not tolerate the proximity of other densely foliaged trees, and is frequently found in forests decimated by fire or cleared by logging.

Description: A tree not usually higher than fifty feet, having a straight, cylindrical trunk and a dense, rounded crown. Fairly short-lived, it is notable for the many shoots it puts out. The bark is smooth and gray green with horizontal streaks, later becoming furrowed. Its slender leaves vary in shape from almost round to oval and are more or less toothed with wavy edges, truncated at the base, pointed or slightly rounded at the tip, and supported by laterally flattened leafstalks that allow the foliar laminas to tremble. The leaves of the stolons, gray and furlike, have a triangular or heartshaped form. The female flowers of this dioecious species are composed of catkins about 3 inches long, whose stigmas are red, silky in texture, and pendent. The male flowers are green, pendent, and 4 to 5 inches long, with light purple anthers. Aspen flowers from February through March.

Qualities:

- Courage
- Intuition
- Inspiration
- Grounding in reality
- Comprehension of the spiritual worlds, accompanied by trust and a sense of protection
- Faith in oneself

Indicated for: those who feel imprisoned by unconscious and inexplicable fears, individuals whose emotional bodies seem hypersensitive and constantly on the alert, so that they live in a state of fearful presentiment. The conscious mind has difficulty making sense of such sensations, so fear, anxiety, restlessness, and anguish are born. People who need Aspen live in a continual state of apprehension without perceiving its underlying cause, which remains veiled. Some danger is glimpsed or foreseen, a vague shadow whose movement is mistaken for reality. This condition acts as a sort of receiving antenna, tuned to pick up environmental conflict and collective psychic disturbances. The ego becomes burdened with fears: of death, darkness, sleeping alone, the threat of war, the economic and political situation, abuse, violence, or monsters and spirits. Aspen children may be frightened of large animals, fairy tales, and witches, or the new teacher at school; they are often anxious and fearful, keeping much to themselves.

I feel protected by my guardian angel.
I open myself to the experiences of life.
I am ready to confront my hidden fears.
I am discovering my inner guide, who overflows with light.

The Skin Zones of Aspen

A   Nasal zone: extends from the midpoint of the eyebrows down the center of the nose to its tip and around its base, covering the whole right side of the nose.
Massage: *light*.

B   Chin zone: extends from the bottom edge of the lower lip and the sides of the mouth to the rim of the chin.
Massage: *light*.

C   Zone above the right collarbone: extends from the side margin of the trapezius and along the upper edge of the collarbone from the shoulder to the base of the neck.
Massage: *light*.

D   Anterior and bilateral shoulder zone: extends 1 inch in diameter over the scapulohumeral articulation on the front of both shoulders.
Massage: *light*.

E   Right parasternal zone: extends ⅜ inch in diameter at the level of the fourth intercostal space.
Massage: *light*.

F   Zone above the left kneecap: area ⅜ inch in diameter over the upper edge of the kneecap and 2 finger widths to the left of its axis.
Massage: *strong*.

G   Zone on the front of the left leg: area ⅜ inch in diameter, 1 finger width in front of the lateral line, and 4 inches above the bimalleolar line of the ankle.
Massage: *light*.

H   Zone on the inner front right leg: area ⅜ inch in diameter, 3 inches above the ankle bone and ⅛ inch in front of the lateral line.
Massage: *light*.

I   Zone on the top of the right foot: area ⅜ inch in diameter located 2 finger widths under the articular line of the foot and ⅜ inch to the outside of its axis.
Massage: *light.*

J   Zone on the right side of the back: rectangular area beginning at the right shoulder blade and covering the end of the clavicle, extending from the second to the fifth dorsal vertebra.
Massage: *light.*

K   Right buttock zone: area 1 inch in diameter at the level of the center of the right buttock.
Massage: *light.*

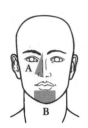

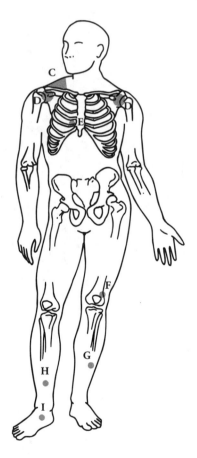

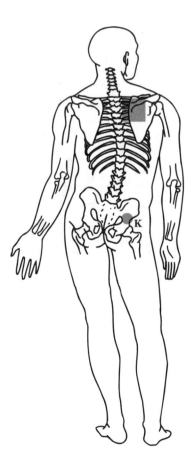

ASPEN

3
Beech
Fagus sylvatica (European Beech)

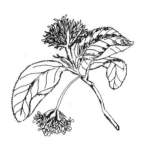

Family: Fagaceae

Habitat: Native to southern and central Europe, where it grows in diversified mountain forests at altitudes up to 6,500 feet. Introduced to North America in the northeast and Pacific states. Beech thrives in cool, deep, relatively dry, well-drained soils.

Description: A tree that can reach over 100 feet in height, 5 feet in diameter, and 300 years of age. The trunk is straight and cylindrical, with smooth, light gray bark that protects the tree from an excess of sun by reflecting ultraviolet rays. The crown is dense and oval in shape. The leaves are alternate, oval, ciliated, and entire, undulate at the edges, short-stemmed, dark green on the right side and lighter green on the underside. Beech is a monoecious tree. Its male inflorescence consists of a short, roundish, pendent catkin bearing clusters of flowers. The male flower is composed of a fused perianth forming a kind of six-pointed bell. The female inflorescence is erect, composed of two flowers inside a prickly husk with four sections, in which the seeds are formed. Winter buds are narrow, long, pointed, and brown. Dead leaves may persist on lower branches throughout the winter. Beech flowers from April through June.

Qualities:

❧ Tolerance
❧ Acceptance

- Compassion for others' imperfections and differences
- Recognition of one's own boundaries
- Inner security
- Self-integration
- Perception of unity within the multiple manifestations of life

Indicated for: extremely critical people who formulate every opinion according to very rigid criteria. They are unable to observe themselves in a spirit of harmony and love, almost as if they did not wish to see that which the inner self suggests by means of the soul's impulse.

Suffering from an inward disharmony, they feel inferior, and so are prone to a sense of vulnerability and insecurity. Closing the door on their inner life, they open their door to the world and observe everything that happens there through the lens of perfectionism, harvesting details with the hypercritical eye of one who exacts perfection and precision. They become intolerant of the lapses and errors of others, and fussiness is the weapon with which they punish those of whom they disapprove. No matter what the cost, they follow their ideals, which they consider the only true ones; they are so convinced of this that they become rigid in the execution of their principles.

This rigidity may manifest itself in aches and pains, particularly rheumatic pains, and in children through awkwardness of movement—they seem to be made of ice. In games it is always the Beech child who makes up the rules, and he is often quite a bully about it, too.

---

*I harvest the harmony of diversity
in myself and others.
I immerse myself in the flow of life.
I perceive my unity with the world.*

Skin Zones of Beech

A   Zone over the right jawbone: begins at a line horizontal to the right corner of the mouth, following the lower margin of the jaw. The front border is formed by a vertical line through the outer corner of the eyebrow and the back border by the jawbone. Massage: *light*.

B   Zone on the upper left of the forehead: area ⅜ inch in diameter. Massage: *strong*.

C   Epigastric zone: oval area with its center at the level of point CV12. Massage: *light*.

D   Right inguinal zone: area 1 inch in diameter located at the level of the upper right groin. Massage: *light*.

E   Left palm zone: area ⅜ inch in diameter in the middle of the inner base of the thumb. Massage: *light*.

F   Left palm zone: rectangular area covering the third finger and the palm down to the line of the wrist. Massage: *light*.

G   Left palm zone: area ⅜ inch in diameter located on the hypothenar eminence, 1 finger width beneath the fold of the wrist in line with the little finger. Massage: *light*.

H   Left leg zone: rectangular area on the medial side of the left leg extending from the popliteal to the middle of the calf. Massage: *light*.

I   Posterior bilateral shoulder zone: area 1 inch in diameter on the posterior axillary line of both the left and right shoulders. Massage: *light*.

J Zone on the right side of the back: rectangular area delineated by the horizontal lines passing through the point and middle of the scapula and extending vertically from the prolongation of the clavicle to the front of the armpit.
Massage: *light.*

K Lumbosacral zone: extends for about 1½ inches to the right and left of the line of the lower spinal vertebrae.
Massage: *light.*

L Zone on the back of the left hand: area ⅜ inch in diameter, in line with the little finger, halfway between the interdigital space and the fold of the wrist.
Massage: *strong.*

M Zone on the back of the left hand: area covering the second finger and the middle of the third finger, extending to the middle of the back of the left hand.
Massage: *light.*

N Zone on the back of the left leg: rectangular area about 1½ inches long, extending from the popliteal to the middle of the left calf.
Massage: *light.*

O Zone on the back of the left leg: area ⅜ inch in diameter located ¾ inch beneath the middle of the left leg and 1 finger width to the outside of its axis.
Massage: *light.*

P Zone on the back of the right leg: area 1 inch in diameter just above the tendon of the Achilles' heel.
Massage: *light.*

Q Zone on the outer side of the right leg: area ⅜ inch in diameter in the middle of the right leg, ¼ inch behind the lateral line.
Massage: *strong.*

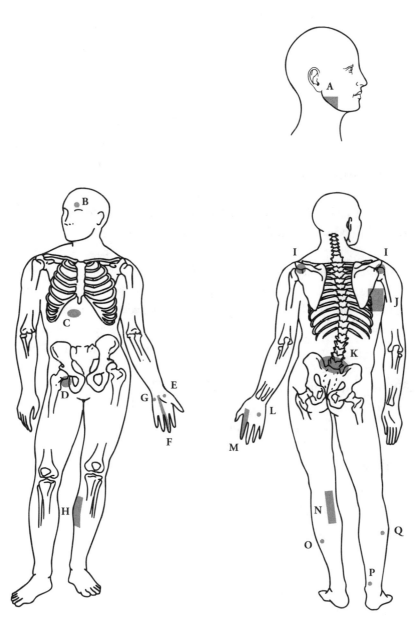

Beech

4
Centaury
Centaurium umbellatum

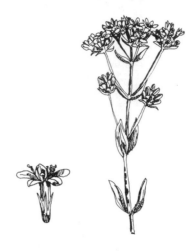

Family: Gentianaceae

Habitat: Europe, from mountainous regions to the seacoast. It is most commonly found in cool, humid, grassy locations.

Description: Annual, herbaceous, hairless, upright plant from 4 to 10 inches high. The stalk is straight and branches at the top into smaller, erect, wide open stems. The basal leaves, oval in shape, are arranged in a rosetta formation; the stemmed leaves are opposite and sessile. The flowers are hermaphroditic and are numerous, small, pink, star-shaped, regular, and sessile, growing from the top of their stems and from the main stalk in dense clusters. The calyx is gamosepalous and the corolla is a straight, cylindrical, greenish white tube. Centaury flowers from June to September.

Qualities:

- Recognition of one's own identity
- Self-determination
- Self-actualization
- Appreciation of one's own willpower
- Self-respect
- Ability to remain true to oneself in a group
- Ability to say "no"

Indicated for: persons so highly sensitive that they can perceive what those around them are feeling and thinking. Their solar plexus is wide open so that the outer world pulls them in all directions, causing them to lose willpower. Their eagerness to serve can amount to a kind of slavery, and they will relinquish their own lives to the office, or to their family or career. They push themselves past their physical limits to better serve others, but their real goal is to receive recognition and acceptance, for they wish at all costs to be "good."

Centaury people register the needs of others without acknowledging their own, giving of themselves unstintingly in order to satisfy their peers. As they have never learned to say "no," any request, no matter the hardship it entails, is readily granted. They are so anxious not to cause disputes or stir up controversy that their availability and servitude create a false persona.

At times they may be attracted to religious cults or political groups, allowing themselves to be molded by the will and influence of teachers, gurus, or politicians. In such cases they submit to the rituals of the group, running the risk of losing their own individuality and precluding the path of personal growth. Ostensibly they accept a given situation, even when they do not entirely share its assumptions.

I acknowledge my identity and inner needs.
I am responsible for the choices I have made of my own will.
I respect and value myself and am responsible for my own
personal development.

Skin Zones of Centaury

A   Left cheek zone: begins at a horizontal line at the bottom of the left side of the nose and ends at a horizontal line at the left corner of the mouth. The inner margin lies on a curved line from the nose to the corner of the mouth, and the outer margin is formed by a vertical line running through the left corner of the left eyebrow. Massage: *light*.

B   Left occipital zone: 1-inch-wide area starting at point GB20 and stretching from the top of the left ear to the lower edge of the skull. The front border lies 2 finger widths behind the left ear. Massage: *light*.

C   Right parietal zone: begins 1½ finger widths to the right of the head's midline, ending 3 finger widths above the tip of the right ear. The back border is aligned vertically with the tip of the ear and extends 3 finger widths forward from that point. Massage: *light*.

D   Zone on the inner left elbow: area ⅜ inch in diameter and 1 finger width above the inner fold of the left elbow. Massage: *light*.

E   Bilateral femoral zone: area 1 inch in diameter located at the level of the top of the thighbone on the lateral line of the body on both the left and right sides. Massage: *light*.

F   Right inguinal-pubic zone: extends from the lower edge of the pubic bone to 1 finger width below an imaginary line from the fold of the buttock to the front, encompassing the genitals. The inner border, formed by the body's midline, extends 4 finger widths to the right. Massage: *light*.

G   Zone on the front left thigh: area 1 inch in diameter, located 4 finger widths above the upper edge of the left kneecap. Massage: *light*.

H   Zone on the front left leg: rectangular area beginning at the horizontal line running through the middle of the shin to its lower quarter. Massage: *light*.

I Zone on the front left leg: area ⅜ inch in diameter, located 4 inches above the bimalleolar line and 1 finger width to the front of the lateral line.
Massage: *light.*

J Right buttock zone: area a little over 2 inches in height, extending from just above the femoral articulation to the right median axillary line.
Massage: *light.*

K Right buttock zone: area 1 inch in diameter, located at the center of the right buttock.
Massage: *light.*

L Right palm zone: area covering the third finger and half of the fourth finger and extending straight down the palm to the fold of the wrist.
Massage: *light.*

M Right leg zone: extending horizontally from the axial line on the back of the right calf outward to the side and front of the leg, and vertically from the middle of the calf to the lower quarter of the leg.
Massage: *light.*

N Zone on the right side of the back: rectangular area extending vertically from the paravertebral line upward to the spine of the posterior clavicle, and horizontally through the lower tip and middle of the scapula.
Massage: *light.*

O Zone on the left side of the back: area located at the level of the third thoracic vertebra on the median line.
Massage: *light.*

P Zone on the right side of the back: area ⅜ inch in diameter and 1 finger width from the median vertebral line, passing horizontally 2 finger widths under the fold of the armpit.
Massage: *light.*

Q Lumbosacral zone: extends for about 1½ inches to the left and right of the line of the lower vertebrae.
Massage: *light.*

R Right foot zone: covers the entire sole of the right foot.
Massage: *light.*

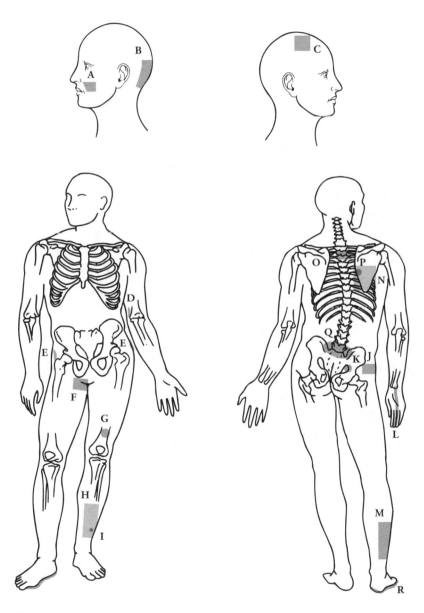

CENTAURY

5
Cerato
Ceratostigma willmottiana

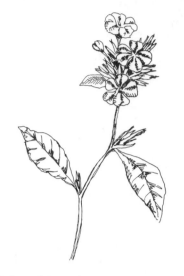

Family: Plumbaginaceae

Habitat: Native to western China, widely cultivated as an ornamental plant elsewhere.

Description: Shrublike plant reaching 5 feet in height. The leaves are deciduous, rhomboid, pointed at the tip, and dark green in color. The flowers are small, deep blue, and tubulous with 5 flattened terminal lobes joined to terminal and axillary racemes. Cerato flowers from July through September.

Qualities:

- Ability to listen to the inner voice
- Inner certainty
- Faith in one's own inner knowledge
- Inspiration
- Coordination of abstract and concrete thinking
- Stimulation of the decision-making process
- Wisdom

Indicated for: persons who are sensitive and intuitive yet lack faith in themselves due to the discrepancy between what they experience on an inner level and what they feel coming at them from the outer world. Because of this they are continually asking others what they should do and how they should behave. Although they know the answer on an intuitive level, they do not accept it on a rational level. It is almost as though they refuse the suggestions springing from the inner voice.

Cerato people seek the solution to their problems by looking to the outer world, to laws and doctrines and the experiences of other people. They accumulate knowledge and experience, but in a passive, sterile way, living by convention and according to counsels and modes of being which they accept in appearance only, even when they put them into practice.

As children they require constant confirmation of what they are doing from parents and teachers, and tend to imitate the games of others rather than create their own.

People in need of Cerato live by reflecting the outer world within themselves. They lack the courage to take individual action or to listen to the voice of intuition.

I follow my intuition, my inner voice.
I have the courage to make decisions based on what I am
inwardly feeling.
I am rediscovering the unity of intuition and rational thought.

SKIN ZONES OF CERATO

A   Left temporal zone: rectangular area beginning at the level of the hairline and ending at the outer corner of the left eyebrow, extending 2½ finger widths to the back of the head.
Massage: *light.*

B   Anterior bilateral shoulder zone: area 1 inch in diameter located at the level of the scapulohumeral articulation on both the left and the right shoulders.
Massage: *light.*

C Right thoracic zone: area ⅜ inch in diameter located on the median axial line, 3 finger widths below the fold of the armpit.
Massage: *light.*

D Left thoracic zone: rectangular area about 3 finger widths in height, beginning at the inner edge of the left side of the rib cage at the level of the xiphoid process, and extending horizontally to the median axial line.
Massage: *light.*

E Left inner elbow zone: area ⅜ inch in diameter and 1 finger width above the inner fold of the left elbow, on the internal lateral line.
Massage: *light.*

F Bilateral femoral zone: area 1 inch in diameter located at the level of the top of both the right and left femur, on the lateral line of the body.
Massage: *light.*

G Zone on the back of the right hand: covers the interdigital space and the two inner halves of the middle and index fingers, running down the back of the right hand to the fold of the wrist.
Massage: *light.*

H Left thigh zone: area 1 inch in diameter located 4 finger widths above the upper edge of the left kneecap.
Massage: *light.*

I Left palm zone: area ⅜ inch in diameter located between the axial line of the middle finger and the third interdigital space, and ⅜ inch beneath the division of the fingers.
Massage: *strong.*

J Left knee zone: area ⅜ in diameter located above the upper edge of the left kneecap and 2 finger widths to the outside of its axis.
Massage: *strong.*

K Bilateral medial knee zone: area 1 inch in diameter located on the median line and on the medial side of both the left and right knees.
Massage: *light.*

L Left shin zone: area ⅜ inch in diameter and about 4 inches above the bimalleolar line and 1 finger width in front of the lateral line on the front of the left leg.
Massage: *light.*

M Right arm-forearm zone: long rectangular area on the medial side of the right upper arm and forearm, passing through the trochlea and extending from the armpit down to the upper quarter of the forearm.
Massage: *light.*

N Zone on the right side of the back: rectangular area extending vertically from the ninth to the eleventh vertebra and horizontally from the paravertebral line to the median axial line.
Massage: *light.*

O Right buttock zone: area 1 inch in diameter located at the center of the right buttock.
Massage: *light.*

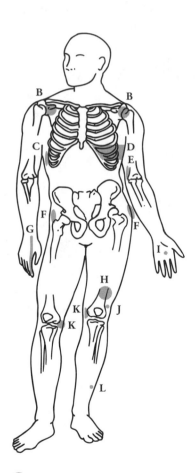
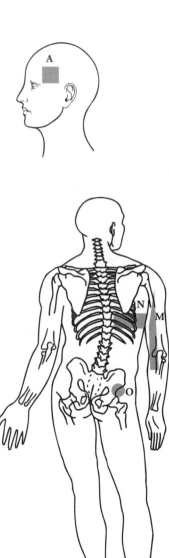

CERATO

6
Cherry Plum
Prunus cerasifera

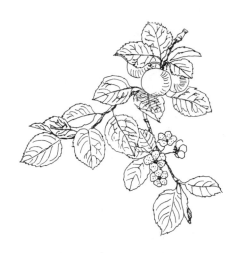

Family: Rosaceae

Habitat: Native to southwest Asia and long cultivated throughout most of Europe, where it has been naturalized for over two thousand years. Naturalized locally in southeast Canada and the eastern and northwestern United States. Also known as "Wild Dwarf Cherry" or "Sour Cherry," Cherry Plum grows along roadsides and fences and in mixed forests at elevations up to 5,900 feet.

Description: A small tree not more than 6 to 8 feet in height with the appearance of a bushy shrub and thin, divaricate, and somewhat drooping branches. Its leaves are ovate to elliptical and not very broad, with sawtoothed edges, smooth and hairless on both sides, and green and shiny on the upper side. Its hermaphroditic flowers are white and peduncled, a little less than 1 inch in diameter, with 5 petals arranged in umbels. Characteristic to this tree is the presence of leaves inside the flowering buds. Cherry Plum flowers from April through May.

Qualities:

- The capacity to live here and now, trusting in life
- Tranquility
- Openness
- Relaxation
- Openness to one's own evolutionary process

- Being oneself
- Harmony between positive and negative polarities within the Self

Indicated for: persons who are afraid of losing control of themselves and committing some horrible action from one moment to the next. Such individuals perceive the destructive forces that exist in each of us and are afraid of them, unable to understand that every process of development, whether mental or spiritual, is based on the seesaw of opposites and the balance between positive and negative forces. They perceive the pole of negative forces with enormous sensibility and, instead of mastering it, they succumb to it. To keep from committing an error they become maniacal perfectionists, always precise for fear of making mistakes or of not being "normal." They may fixate on things or create obsessions for themselves to the point of psychosis.

As children they exhibit repetitive behaviors leading to self-isolation and even autism, often pacing back and forth, clapping their hands, or slamming the door. They do not listen to what their parents say, yet they manage to control themselves and can be "perfect" children—in their rooms everything is put away in its proper place, folded and entirely in order. Suddenly, however, they can have violent reactions of rage if they find themselves unable to control a situation.

I integrate the opposing poles of life within myself.
I open my luminous self to the evolutionary process and I progress in tranquility.
I surrender myself to the inner guide with openness and love.

SKIN ZONES OF CHERRY PLUM

A   Right ear zone: area 3 inches in diameter located at the level of the earlobe on the outer face of the auricular pavilion.
Massage: *strong*.

B Cervical zone: oval area on the median line located at the level of the seventh cervical vertebra.
Massage: *light.*

C Left hip zone: rectangular area above the left buttock, extending from the fifth lumbar to the second sacral vertebra and from the paravertebral line to the posterior axial line.
Massage: *light.*

D Lumbosacral zone: extends for about 1½ inches to both the right and left of the line of the lower vertebrae.
Massage: *light.*

E Right buttock zone: area 1 inch in diameter located in the center of the right buttock.
Massage: *light.*

F Right thoracic zone: area ⅜ inch in diameter and 3 finger widths from the fold of the armpit on the median line.
Massage: *light.*

G Right thoracic zone: area on the front of the right shoulder, 4 finger widths above the fold of the armpit and just below the collarbone.
Massage: *strong.*

H Left hip zone: area located at the level of the anterior inferior iliac spine and 2 finger widths from the lateral line of the body on the front of the left hip.
Massage: *strong.*

I Bilateral wrist zone: oval area over the median line on the inner wrist of each arm.
Massage: *light.*

J Right thigh zone: rectangular area on the front of the right thigh 3 inches beneath the horizontal line passing through the center of the groin.
Massage: *light.*

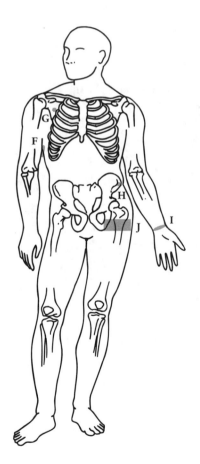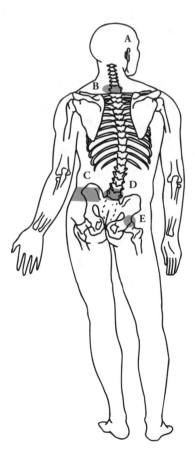

CHERRY PLUM

7
Chestnut Bud
Aesculus hippocastanum (Horsechestnut)

Family: Hippocastanaceae

Habitat: Originally native to southeastern Europe in the Caucasus and the Balkans, introduced in western and northern Europe in the sixteenth century, and widely planted throughout North America, it now grows wild in the northeastern United States.

Description: A large, elegant, short-lived tree up to 75 feet in height with a dense, regular, rounded crown. The bark is a dark reddish or grayish color and flakes off in big scaly plates. The palmate, compound leaves are opposite and carried on a long, rough stalk. They form a fan shape as 7 to 9 wedge-shaped, toothed, unequal leaflets radiating from a common point. The buds are large and very sticky. The large bisexual flowers have bilateral symmetry and are white, spotted red and yellow at the base, and borne in conical, upright, branched clusters. The calyx has 4 unequal teeth; the corolla has 4 unequal and undulate petals; there are 7 to 9 stamens and 1 protruding style; and the ovary is divided into 3 lobes. The familiar shiny brown nuts are found within the three-part green husk.

    Caution: *These nuts are poisonous and must not be eaten, as they contain a dangerous glycoside.*

Qualities:

    ⇗ Capacity to process experience in a constructive way
    ⇗ Learning

- Clarity of vision before one's own errors and negative experiences, in order to avoid their repetition
- Clarity of ideas
- Ability to live in the present
- Capacity to change with clarity
- Ability to benefit from experience

Indicated for: those who cannot manage to coordinate their inner worlds with reality and its flow. Since they are unable to assess the relationship between these two worlds, the inner self cannot learn from lived experience. These people derive no benefits from experience, as they never allow it to mature under the inner sun. They seem not to want to conclude a cycle in order to begin a new one, and instead spin like tops, prey to the next glamorous fantasy about the future. They keep tripping over the same mistakes, as they are unaware of having made them already, and, rather than realizing the actual moment, they live in projections of the future, where they need not carry any experiential baggage. They may lack concentration and pay scant attention to the present, all the while wishing for "tomorrow," and live with their heads in the clouds, forgetting what they had to do today.

As children they repeat the same actions every day in a mechanical manner: they repeatedly forget the same notebook; they can't work through errors they made the day before because they don't remember having made them; they are unable to hold on to experiences and nurture them to maturity.

I learn from my mistakes
and make of them an inner treasure.
I live in a present rich with past experience.
Experiences are the fruits of my existence.

SKIN ZONES OF CHESTNUT BUD

A   Right arm zone: area ⅜ inch in diameter on the front of the upper right arm, located 2 finger widths under the armpit between the external lateral and ventral axial lines.
Massage: *strong.*

B   Right thoracic zone: area ⅜ inch in diameter and 3 finger widths under the fold of the armpit on the median line.
Massage: *light.*

C   Left arm zone: area ⅜ inch in diameter and 2 finger widths above the fold of the elbow on the inner side of the left arm.
Massage: *light.*

D   Bilateral femoral zone: area 1 inch in diameter, located on the lateral line of the body at the level of the top of the femur on both the left and right legs.
Massage: *light.*

E   Right thigh zone: rectangular area beginning on a horizontal line, extending 1 finger width below the fold of the right buttock, and ending 1 finger width above the kneecap. The upper end is 4 finger widths from the midline of the body; the lower end of the inner border lies 2 finger widths to the left of the right kneecap.
Massage: *light.*

F   Left thigh zone: area 1 inch in diameter located 4 finger widths above the upper edge of the left kneecap.
Massage: *light.*

G   Cervical zone: oval area on the axial line at the level of the seventh cervical vertebra.
Massage: *light.*

H   Left popliteal zone: area 1 inch in diameter at the center of the popliteal cave at the back of the left knee.
Massage: *light.*

I   Right calf zone: rectangular, 2-inch-wide area on the back of the right leg beginning 4 finger widths above the upper margin of the inner ankle bone and ending 6 finger widths above that. The back border runs up the middle of the calf on a line that extends from the Achilles tendon to the middle of the knee.

Massage: *light.*

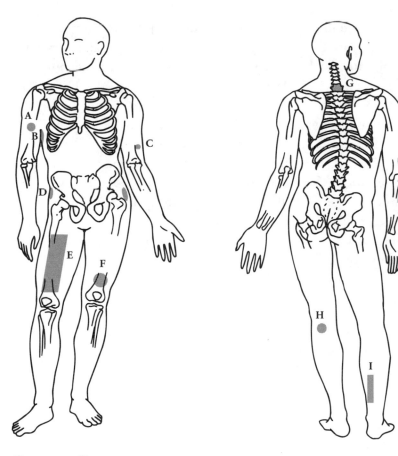

CHESTNUT BUD

8
Chicory
Cichorium intybus

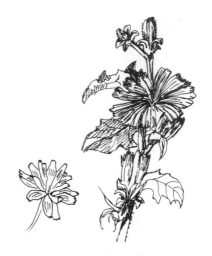

Family: Compositae

Habitat: Common throughout Europe except in the northern countries. Chicory thrives in dry, clayey soils rich in lime and is found in uncultivated fields throughout plains, hillsides, and mountains at elevations up to 5,000 feet.

Description: Annual, biennial, or perennial herb with a robust taproot. The stalk is rigid, angular, and furry, with multiple branchings. The lower leaves are deeply and sharply toothed and rather elongate; the top leaves sheathe the stem and are small, elongate, pubescent, with deep lobes. The flowers are borne on annual, erect stems 5 feet or less in height. They are bright blue in color, 1 to 1 ½ inches wide, furnished with ligules and 5 stamens concrescible with anthers. Chicory flowers from July to September.

Qualities:

- Unconditional love
- Giving without expectation of recompense
- Self-nourishment without dependence
- Archetypal motherhood
- Devotion
- Warmth
- Protection and security to others
- Respect for others' freedom

Indicated for: those who suffer from a profound inner dissatisfaction because they do not feel truly loved and accepted by the world. They suffer from an inner sense of insecurity, linked to the fear of losing someone or something. They may become extremely protective of their children, meddling in family affairs and trying to intervene in decisions and organize, guide, advise, and decide even in those situations that do not concern them.

This possessive attitude on the part of the personality manifests itself in forms of emotional bribery such as loving in order to get something back, maintaining a friendship for reasons of personal egotism, and doing something for someone else in order to receive something.

Chicory people live in a world of ifs: "I'll love you if . . . ; I'll give you a kiss if . . . ; I'll give you some money if . . . ; I'm old and I'll give you the house if . . . ; I've loved you all my life in exchange for . . . ." Insecurity is joined to possessiveness, a tendency to oppress and dominate, and a sort of greediness, a desire for recompense due.

As children they believe that everything belongs to them. Outrageously possessive, they live in a continual process of extortion and bribery: "I'll do this *if*." They are overattached to their mothers and frequently jealous. Chicory children, particularly girls, may suffocate their dolls with cuddles and caresses, excessive attention and tendernesses—the prelude to a stifling love.

❧❧❧

I live in unconditional, universal love.
I am accepted in the world as a living being.
I give unconditionally to the entire world.

❧❧❧

Skin Zones of Chicory

A   Right periorbital zone: extends from the lower edge of the eyebrow down to the lower edge of the eye socket. The inner border aligns with the inside edge of the iris, and the outside border

aligns with the outer tip of the eyebrow.
Massage: *light.*

B Right parietal zone: square area beginning at the upper edge of the right ear and extending 3 finger widths upward. The front border aligns vertically with the tip of the ear; the zone extends 3 finger widths backward.
Massage: *light.*

C–D Bilateral shoulder zone: area 1 inch in diameter located on the front of both the left and right shoulders at the level of the scapulohumeral articulation.
Massage: *light.*

E Right iliac zone: area 1 inch in diameter over the right iliac fossa, under the horizontal line passing through the middle of the umbilical-pubic line.
Massage: *light.*

F Bilateral wrist zone: oval area on the axial line on both the left and right inner arms.
Massage: *light.*

G Left thigh zone: rectangular area occupying almost the entire front of the left thigh, from the line above the kneecap to 3 finger widths under the groin.
Massage: *light.*

H Right thigh zone: area 1 inch in diameter located on the front of the right thigh just above the top of the kneecap.
Massage: *light.*

I Right leg zone: area ⅜ inch in diameter located on the front of the right leg ¾ inch to the inside of the axial line and 2 finger widths beneath the lower edge of the kneecap.
Massage: *light.*

J Left lower leg zone: rectangular area beginning 3½ finger widths below the left kneecap and extending downward 6 finger widths, with side borders that lie 2 finger widths to the left and right side

of the kneecap.
Massage: *light.*

K Zone on the left side of the back: area ⅜ inch in diameter located
over the iliovertebral angle on the left side of the lower back in
line with the tip of the left elbow.
Massage: *light.*

L Left forearm zone: area on the back of the left forearm extending
from the fold of the wrist halfway up the forearm.
Massage: *light.*

M Left lower leg zone: area ⅜ inch in diameter located on the back
of the left calf, ⅝ inch beneath the middle of the leg and 1 finger
width to the outside of the axial line.
Massage: *light.*

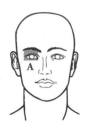

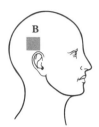

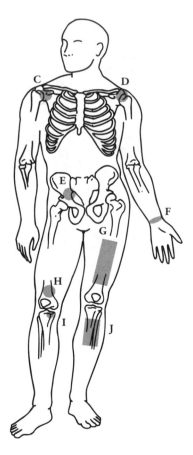

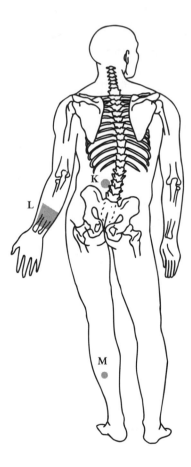

CHICORY

9
Clematis
Clematis vitalba

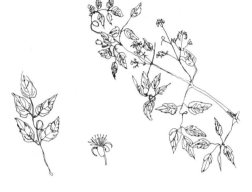

Family: Ranunculaceae

Habitat: Thrives in thickets, woodland undergrowth, and the edges of woods, in plains, on hillsides, and in mountainous regions up to 5,000 feet in Europe.

Description: A vine that can live as long as 25 years and reach a length of 65 feet, taking on a shrublike appearance as it ages. Its climbing stem is woody, angular, and vigorous and clings by its leafstems. The leaves are green, opposite, and pinnate, composed of 3 to 9 toothed leaflets, which can be oval, pointed, or heart-shaped. The flowers, borne in branching inflorescences, have a diameter of 20 millimeters and are white, without petals. Their 4 wooly sepals are arranged in a cross and have numerous stamens. Clematis flowers from June to August.

Qualities:

- ➤ Grounded in life
- ➤ Creative idealism fulfilled
- ➤ Concrete actualization
- ➤ Anchored in the present
- ➤ Harmony of life in the present
- ➤ Expression of one's perceptions in the material world

Indicated for: those who seem to live another life, in another world built exclusively for them—a world of dreams and imagination, where everything seems beautiful and good.

Such people may talk with you yet seem to be elsewhere, thinking of something else; they cannot seem to muster up much interest for what is happening in the present. They create illusions to such a point that the world appears to them to move along the lines of their fantastic constructions. Their memory is often poor and their visual and auditory perceptions are capable of creating unreal sounds and images, while they react indifferently to events in the real world. Clematis people may have great intuitions, but these will remain relegated to the world of imagination without ever being translated into reality.

They may be so distracted as to seem clumsy; they frequently trip, bump into things, and knock things over. In a restaurant they are apt to bump carelessly into the waiter, knocking the tray of plates out of his hand.

Clematis children have their heads in the clouds. While the teacher is explaining the subject at hand, they are watching the butterflies outside, creating imaginary beings out of pieces of paper. They seem not to hear or be able to focus on the words written up on the blackboard.

*I actualize the projects of my imagination
in the material world.
I channel myself into the flow of the world.
I participate in the present, constructing
it in tangible ways and relinquishing
my attachment to what is vague and indeterminate.*

SKIN ZONES OF CLEMATIS

A   Right zygomatic arch zone: area beginning at the level of the right orbit and ending at a horizontal line at the lower edge of the nose in line with its tip. The outside margin aligns with the outer tip of the right eyebrow and the inside margin lies about 1 finger width from the nose. Massage: *light*.

B   Right retromandibular zone: square area extending between the mastoid and the temperomanibular joint.
Massage: *light.*

C   Right arm zone: area ⅜ inch in diameter and 2 finger widths below the armpit, between the ventral axial line and the external lateral line.
Massage: *strong.*

D   Right thoracic zone: area ⅜ in diameter and 3 finger widths below the fold of the armpit on the median line.
Massage: *light.*

E   Right abdominal zone: area ⅜ inch in diameter and 3 finger widths above and to the right of the navel.
Massage: *strong.*

F   Inner left arm zone: area ⅜ inch in diameter and 2 finger widths above the fold of the elbow, lying just to the outside of the axial line on the inner side of the left arm.
Massage: *light.*

G   Bilateral femoral zone: area 1 inch in diameter on the lateral line of the body at the level of the top of the femur on both the left and right hip.
Massage: *light.*

H   Bilateral foot zone: area ⅜ inch in diameter located at the level of Sp2 on both the left and right foot.
Massage: *light.*

I   Right leg zone: area ⅜ inch in diameter located on the back of the right calf on the horizontal line at the middle of the leg and just to the right of the lateral line.
Massage: *light.*

J   Left foot zone: aligns horizontally with the upper edge of the left ankle bone, extending downward to cover the foot and half of the heel. Its back border is formed by the Achilles tendon. The front border begins at the back edge of the outer ankle bone and slopes gently frontward.
Massage: *light.*

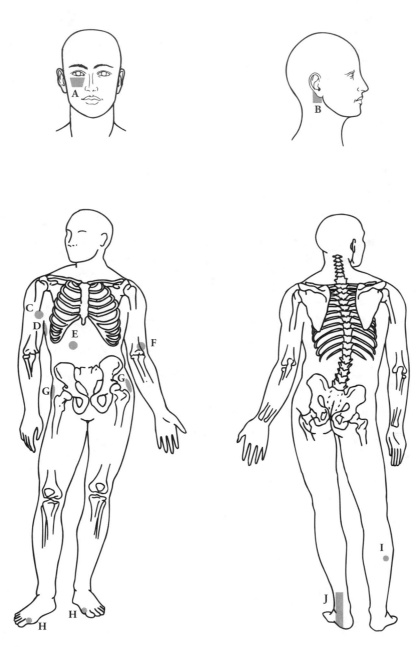

CLEMATIS

10
Crab Apple
Malus pumila

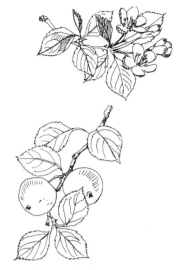

Family: Rosaceae

Habitat: Found in Europe in the mixed deciduous forests of plains, hills, and mountains up to 3,200 feet and often associated with oak, beech, chestnut, and maple.

Description: A tree that rarely exceeds 50 feet in height, the crab apple often gives the appearance of a large bush with extremely dense branches, some of which turn into thorns after the terminal bud has fallen. The bark is a dark gray brown, irregularly furrowed, and falls away in scales. The leaves, supported on rather short stems, are oval, serrated at the edges, plushly hairy, and gray. The highly perfumed flowers are borne at the tip of the twigs in clusters and have roundish petals, about 1 inch long, which are white with deep red interiors; the anthers of their numerous stamens are yellow. Crab apple flowers from April through May.

Qualities:

- Purification
- Order
- Improvement
- Acceptance of the imperfect
- Inner cleanliness
- Rebirth

≫ Detoxification
≫ Inner candor

Indicated for: those who feel themselves to be flawed so that they suffer from a continual sensation of uncleanliness, worrying that their sweater may smell of sweat, imagining that their skin is too oily, their hair too greasy, and their breath heavy and unpleasant. Such people are fixated on the idea that they are dirty, even filthy, almost unworthy of belonging to the human race. They are trapped in sensations of chaos and squalor.

People in need of Crab Apple are afraid of dirtying their hands and harbor a fear of insects and animals which could bring infections into the house. Their housecleaning is so meticulous as to be maniacal, and care of the body is greatly exaggerated. They may brush their teeth a dozen times a day, whether they have eaten or not; they cannot bear the wrinkle forming on their forehead, the sunspot that appeared on their temple during the summer, or the visible veins in their hands or legs.

Mentally, they may feel shame for harboring hateful or disagreeable thoughts or experiencing resentment toward a friend. Overall, these individuals feel stained by a false sense of guilt, simply for having materialized on the earth.

Crab apple can also be used to eliminate organic toxins during times of fast, and as a detoxicant after a long course of pharmaceutical drugs. It is equally useful for therapists who have absorbed the negative vibrations transmitted by their clients, and for persons with allergies. It is the flower of choice for all those who manifest their interior conflicts by way of the skin.

I purify myself of evil thoughts.
I accept the reality of an imperfect world.
I am patient with myself and with others on our journey
toward physical and moral perfection.

SKIN ZONES OF CRAB APPLE

A   Left temporal zone: area ⅜ inch in diameter and 1 finger width from the outer tip of the left eyebrow.
Massage: *strong.*

B   Throat zone: area extending from the chin down over the throat and neck, covering the bilateral sternocleidomastoid muscles down to the midpoint of the neck.
Massage: *light.*

C   Left paravertebral zone: extends from the eleventh dorsal vertebra to the fourth lumbar in an area having a width of 2¼ inches.
Massage: *light.*

D   Left thigh zone: area ⅜ inch in diameter located in the middle of the back of the left thigh on the axial line.
Massage: *light.*

E   Inner left arm zone: area ⅜ inch in diameter and 3 finger widths under the fold of the armpit and 1 finger width to the right of the internal lateral line.
Massage: *strong.*

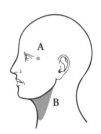

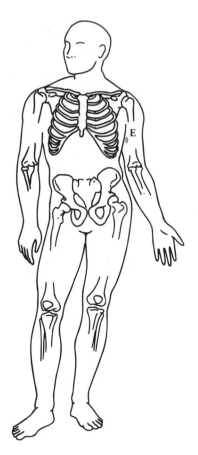

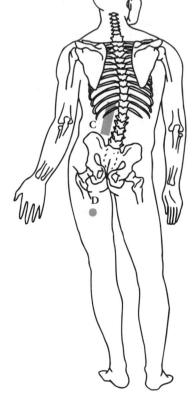

CRAB APPLE

11

Elm

Ulmus procera (English Elm)

Family: Ulmaceae

Habitat: Originally native to the British Isles and a characteristic tree of the English landscape, English Elm has been widely planted in North America since colonial times. Once widespread throughout the countryside, especially along roadways and hedgerows, it is now gravely threatened by Dutch elm disease. Frequently planted along pathways and in gardens as an ornamental, it prefers rich, moist, and very fertile soil.

Description: A large tree that may reach 130 feet in height and 10 feet in diameter, the elm sends out numerous runners and is often surrounded by younger elms. The crown is dense, broad, and rounded, formed by massive, spreading, nearly upright branches positioned high on the trunk. The bark is dark brown and furrowed, forming little rectangular scales. The roundish leaves are alternate, simple, deciduous, double-toothed, more or less pointed at the tip, and clearly asymmetrical at the base. They are a vivid green, somewhat rough on the right side, with a pale down running along the veins on the underside, and are supported on short, hairy stems. The numerous flowers are dark red, hermaphroditic, and almost sessile, arranged in small, alternate bunches. They appear very early, before any leaves. English elm flowers anytime between February and April.

Qualities:

- Responsibility
- Self-confidence
- Leadership abilities
- Capacity to handle situations
- Faith that help will come at the right moment
- Altruism

Indicated for: people who have always been leaders or good at managing, yet who suddenly lose all faith in their abilities. They feel like failures and total incompetents; the world seems to be caving in on them and they don't know why. They are no longer supported by their friends, their partner, or their ideals, and everything becomes very difficult. A desire to abandon everything and everyone reemerges, since they themselves feel abandoned, as though drowning in a sea of chores and commitments. They must face their difficulties and choices alone while feeling inadequate and overburdened with responsibilities.

This flower is also very useful for children who are away from their parents for much of the day, engaged in a hundred different activities: school, swimming, guitar lessons, rehearsals, and so on. Overwhelmed by myriad projects and tasks, incapable of keeping up with it all, they crumble and no longer want to go on.

I have faith in my abilities.
I am doing my best in a difficult situation.
I am never discouraged.

Skin Zones of Elm

A   Bilateral subclavicle zone: area about ½ inch in diameter located just below the outer end of the clavicle on both the left and right

shoulders.
Massage: *light.*

B   Left arm zone: area about 1½ finger widths above the inner fold of the left elbow on the lateral line.
Massage: *light.*

C   Left thigh zone: area about 1 inch in diameter located 4 finger widths above the kneecap on the front of the left thigh.
Massage: *light.*

D   Left knee zone: area just above the upper edge of the left kneecap and 2 finger widths to the outside of the axial line.
Massage: *strong.*

E   Right leg zone: area ⅜ inch in diameter located about 3½ inches above the ankle bone and ⅛ inch in front of the lateral line.
Massage: *light.*

F   Left lateral thoracic zone: area about 1 inch in diameter on the left side of the thorax just under the armpit.
Massage: *light.*

G   Zone on the right side of the back: area ⅜ inch in diameter located on the horizontal plane passing 2 finger widths under the fold of the right armpit and 1 finger width from the median vertebral line.
Massage: *light.*

H   Left thoracic zone: rectangular area extending between the anterior and posterior axial lines from the armpit to the horizontal line passing through the lower point of the scapula.
Massage: *light.*

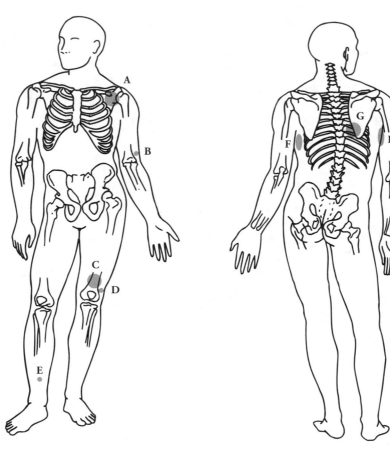

ELM

12

Gentian

Gentiana amarella

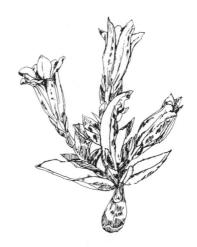

Family: Gentianaceae

Habitat: Gentian grows in Europe in open fields, on heaths and moors, and in sandy soils at elevations up to 5,500 feet.

Description: Biennial plant anywhere between 1 and 20 inches high, made up of a narrow column of short branches with many flowers grouped around the main stalk. The basal rosette is composed of lanceolate or ribbon-shaped leaves that disappear at the beginning of autumn; the second-year basal leaves are invariably lanceolate. The flower is composed of a calyx with long, narrow, triangular teeth and a purple or reddish (rarely white or yellow) corolla, about ⅜ to 1¾ inches long and 5 to 9 inches wide. Gentian flowers from June to October.

Qualities:

- Perseverance
- Ability to overcome adversity
- Trust in life
- Optimism
- Courage
- Confidence in one's own actions
- Dissolution of doubts
- Shining light flowing into depression's darkness
- Faith, an inward belief

Indicated for: persons who are pervaded in every cell by doubt and lack of faith in themselves and in life. Everything that can go wrong manifests in frustrating thoughts of failure and incompetence; the least gesture ends in defeat, since losing is a built-in mental construct. Gentian people are easily discouraged and the smallest difficulty can become insurmountable. They refuse to engage in the trials and challenges of life, and such tests are put off again and again with a thousand excuses. Depression can sneak in and in a short time invade the body to such a degree that the individual may isolate him- or herself from the world, becoming apathetic and indifferent. The physical body swiftly follows the emotional and mental bodies, becoming ever more frequently ill in order to escape an environment and situation that require commitment and work. What is lacking is inner motivation, that faith that nudges us forward in life and leads to fulfillment.

People in need of this flower are out of touch with the enlivening spirit dwelling within us; in their case, the soul is unable to inform the body and transmit to and through it the impulses of spirit. Although they try to overcome this by way of reasoning and logical analysis, things soon fall apart, landing them in a state of discontentment and frustration since they are not vivified by an inward strength or faith.

Children who respond to this remedy are unconsolably dissatisfied and always defeated, so they never initiate a game or bout of playfulness on impulse. Instead, they stand aside and wait for someone else to call them over and infuse them with a little energy and light. Uninterested and apathetic as they are, friends and family must constantly rouse them out of their torpor, involving them in every activity imaginable.

Gentian is also used in cases of chronic illness and convalescence.

I surrender to being enlivened by the spirit.
I persevere in the face of difficulty, illuminating the darkened
path before me.
I have put profound trust in my potential.
I nurture the faith that lives inside me.

Skin Zones of Gentian

A   Left cheek zone: area beginning on a horizontal line on the level of the bottom of the nose and ending at a horizontal line on the level of the left corner of the mouth. The front border is vertically aligned with the outside tip of the left eyebrow, extending back to end at the base of the left earlobe.
Massage: *light.*

B   Bilateral elbow zone: area 1 inch in diameter located on the central part of the inner fold of both the left and right elbows.
Massage: *light.*

C   Left leg zone: area ⅜ inch in diameter and located 4 inches above the bimalleolar line and 1 finger width in front of the lateral line on the front of the lower left leg.
Massage: *light.*

D   Right leg zone: area ⅜ inch in diameter and about 3 inches above the ankle bone and ¼ inch in front of the lateral line on the inner front surface of the lower right leg.
Massage: *light.*

E   Right dorsal zone: large rectangular area located on the median clavicular line from the iliac crest up to the tenth rib on the right side of the back.
Massage: *light.*

F   Right leg zone: area ⅜ inch in diameter located 1 inch below the fold of the popliteal and 1 finger width to the outside of the axial line on the back of the lower right leg.
Massage: *strong.*

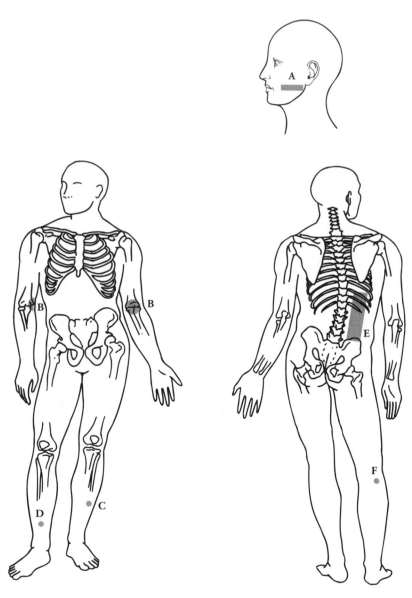

GENTIAN

13
Gorse
Ulex europaeus

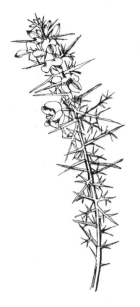

Family: Leguminoseae

Habitat: Native to European heaths and moors, Gorse has been introduced in North America and now grows spontaneously in the Atlantic states and on the West Coast, where its bright yellow flowers cover many coastline cliffs.

Description: An erect, pubescent, 3- to 6-foot-tall, very dense and extremely thorny shrub, whose principal stems, lateral branches, and lanceolate or linear leaves all end in sharp points. The highly perfumed flower is solitary, with a very short stalk. Its dimensions vary from ½ to ¾ inch and it is composed of an intense yellow corolla whose wings are longer than its keel. Gorse flowers from February through June.

Qualities:

- Hope
- Renewed sense of possibility
- Rekindled desire to wrestle with life
- Balanced soul within the polarities of life
- Infusion of inner alchemical light
- Restored life purpose
- Recognition of obstacles in one's path

- Refusal to give up
- Perseverance through hardship

Indicated for: those who live without hope in anything or anyone, who are desperate and resigned and have inwardly given up on the world. The etheric body, living in this state of abandonment, fails to construct the appropriate corporal defenses; everything seems disorganized and each part of the body functions in an autonomous mode, unrelated to the others. Perception of the integrity of the body becomes blurred, so that people end up fixating on and worrying about the health of their heart, their lungs, or their legs. They feel easily exhausted and attacked by obscure forces. Every disorder seems to be bringing them closer to the grave with extreme rapidity. Perhaps they lack the ability to accept life's plan for them, entering into conflict with it rather than allowing it to flower. Everything turns into suffering, nothing has any more purpose, the world is without hope. The person's face sets into sadness, the light in their eyes is quenched, and the expressive facial lines vanish, giving way to the amorphous mask of despair. People in need of gorse complain continually about life itself.

Children who respond to this remedy are listless and immobile and react to suggestions to do things with "Oh, it's no use," or "No, that's okay." They are without expectations, having suffered some physical, mental, or spiritual trauma that has paralyzed them, damming the flow of their inner energies. They appear completely blocked; inside themselves they are on strike, unwilling to go forward. Due to some profound repression, they limit and punish themselves.

I look on the bright side of life.
Hope and joy flow into me.
I accept and fulfill the spiritual plan.
I am born anew, willing to take on the struggles of life.

Skin Zones of Gorse

A   Neck zone: rectangular area on the left side of the neck, beginning at the base of the skull and ending at the base of the neck. The right border is 1½ finger widths to the side of the midline of the neck; the left border is 2 finger widths behind the back of the left ear, extending downward.
Massage: *light.*

B   Right shoulder zone: area ⅜ inch in diameter located 2 finger widths under the acromion and 1 finger width to the inside of the anterior axial line on the front of the right shoulder.
Massage: *strong.*

C   Left forearm zone: oval area located on the inside of the left forearm, beginning 3 finger widths below the fold of the elbow and extending downward toward the wrist for 5 finger widths.
Massage: *light.*

D   Right thigh zone: area 1 inch in diameter located on the upper front right thigh to the outside of the median line of the thigh and just below the right greater trochanter.
Massage: *light.*

E   Bilateral upper arm zone: rectangular area located on the inside of the median line running down the back of both the left and right upper arms, beginning at the bend of the elbow.
Massage: *light.*

F   Left thigh zone: round area 2 inches in diameter located on the posterior median line in the upper third of the back of the left thigh.
Massage: *light.*

G   Right leg zone: area ⅜ inch in diameter located 1 inch below the fold of the knee and 1 finger width to the outside of the median line running down the back of the right leg.
Massage: *strong.*

H Right thigh zone: area ⅜ inch in diameter located 4 inches below the anterior superior iliac spine, on the lateral line of the back of the right thigh.
Massage: *light.*

I Left hand zone: area ⅜ inch in diameter located on the median line of the fourth finger on the back of the left hand, halfway between the fold of the wrist and the base of the finger.
Massage: *light.*

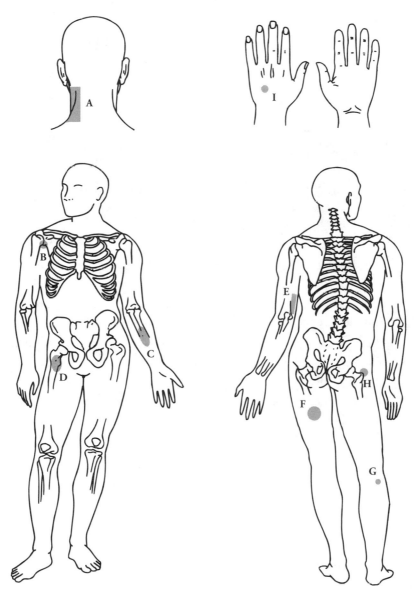

GORSE

14
Heather
Calluna vulgaris (Scotch Heather)

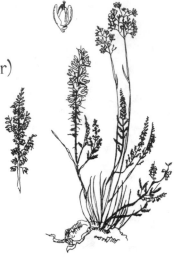

Family: Ericaceae

Habitat: Asia, Europe, Eastern Canada, and in the United States from Michigan to West Virginia. Heather thrives in poor soils, cold to temperate climates, and rainy weather.

Description: A twisted, branching, woody shrub with slender, erect, ascendent branches, varying in height up to 3 feet. Heather can live for as long as 40 years. The leaves are sessile, opposite, and arranged in 4 rows. They are linear, embricate, and obtuse, very small, and elongated at the base so as to form two small, shining, dark green ears. The very numerous small, pink-to-lavender, somewhat pendent flowers, are borne in leafy, unilateral clusters. The corolla is bell-shaped with 4 lobes. Heather flowers from July to October.

Qualities:

- Participation
- Identification with others
- Serenity and interior silence
- Tolerance
- Ability to listen to others
- Empathy
- Ability to listen to the inner self

Indicated for: those who feel isolated from themselves and from others, yet desire to communicate their feelings. This need is so great that they must manifest it at all costs, and they do so by talking. Their emotions overlap and entwine so that they are unable to distinguish one from another. Discussing them is an attempt to put them in some sort of order, yet ends up creating confusion for both speaker and listeners. People in need of Heather will start talking about something but never wrap it up or reach a conclusion, since they lose the thread and slide swiftly from one subject to another. This happens at such a fast pace that by the end of the day the person ends up wondering what he or she has actually said.

Children who respond to this remedy are born attention-getters. Rowdy exhibitionists, they tend to butt in all the time and talk out of place. Because of this peers are likely to avoid them and this sets into motion the mechanisms for Heather individuals' major need for attention. Egocentric because they have not yet perfectly unified their energetic bodies, they feel distance from and lack of integration with their spirit. They are children who are not yet truly grown.

I integrate my physical self in the spirit and begin to mature.
I identify with others and know how to listen.
In silence I listen to the voice of my inner self.

SKIN ZONES OF HEATHER

A   Left frontal zone: area ⅜ inch in diameter on the upper left side of the forehead.
   Massage: *strong.*

B   Left thoracic zone: area between the third and fifth ribs on the inside of the clavicular median line, 1 finger width from the edge of the left side of the sternum.
   Massage: *light.*

C   Right leg zone: area 1 inch above the edge of the inner ankle bone of the right leg.
Massage: *light.*

D   Left palm zone: area ⅜ inch in diameter located at the level of the hypothenar on the interdigital line of the fourth finger, 1 finger width below the fold of the wrist on the left palm.
Massage: *light.*

E   Lumbosacral zone: extends for about 1½ inches to the left and right of the line of the lower spinal vertebrae.
Massage: *light.*

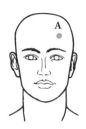
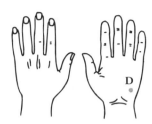
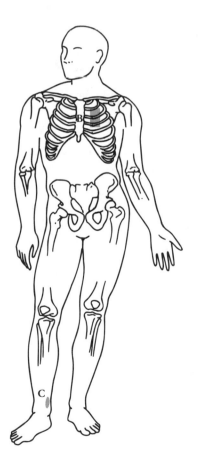
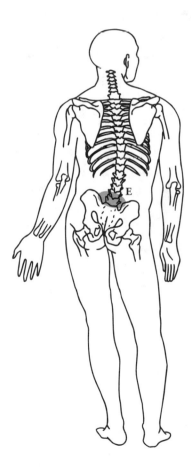

HEATHER

15
Holly
Ilex aquifolium

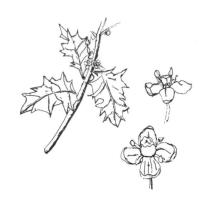

Family: Aquifoliaceae

Habitat: Forests in hilly and mountainous regions up to 6,500 feet.

Description: A tree that may reach 30 feet in height, having persistent leaves, although it is generally encountered as a small shrub in the underbrush of forests. The leaves are simple, stiff, hard, waxy, alternate, dark green above and a light, opaque green underneath. Those on the lower branches are undulate and toothed, bearing sharp thorns on their edges, while those on the higher branches are flat, oval, and entire. The short-stemmed flowers are white or pink, rather hard to see, and arranged in clusters at the axil of the subsessile leaves. Male and female flowers are borne on two different plants, so there are two distinct types of holly, one male and one female. Holly flowers from May through June.

Qualities:

- Unconditional, disinterested, transpersonal love
- Unimpeded flow of love throughout the heart
- Verbal and physical expression of empathy
- Divine love
- Comprehension of the world of human feelings
- Perception of others' love for oneself

- ➤ Universal compassion
- ➤ Perception of the infinite potential of love

Indicated for: those who are inwardly insecure due to abuse of one kind or another, and who feel deprived of the love of their families or partners. They feel rejected by the world, almost as if they had no right to be here. Wherever they look they see adversity and feel that no matter what they do, they will surely be rejected. They become irritable, surly, suspicious, jealous, and dissatisfied and begin to plot their revenge. They start to feel hatred toward their fellow human beings and can explode into violent demonstrations of rage, to the point of fisticuffs.

Their hearts close to the perception of love so that they are unable to nurture their potential. They become sterile, arid as deserts, starving and thirsting and scheming to seek revenge against the entire world. They feel that their bodies are not being nourished by love and are drying out.

Holly is the remedy of choice for children experiencing jealousy of a newborn sibling and for those who were not accepted during pregnancy, suffering in utero rejection. Such children can become violent, quarrelsome, rude, and envious and often break their friends' toys. They live in a continual process of rejection and exclusion from the world.

I am accepted with love by the world.
I explore and express all the potential resources of my love.
In unity with the cosmos, I participate freely and radiate joy.

SKIN ZONES OF HOLLY

A   Bilateral frontal zone: triangular area on each side of the head, beginning on a vertical line 1½ finger widths to the left and right

of the midline of the head and extending 3 finger widths to the sides. The front border lies on the hairline and extends backward 3 finger widths.
Massage: *light.*

B   Bilateral cheek zone: rectangular area beginning at the corner of the mouth and ending at the jaw line on both the left and right cheeks. The front border aligns vertically with the corner of the mouth, the back border with the outer corner of the eyebrow on both sides of the face.
Massage: *light.*

C   Right temporomandibular zone: area beginning just above the right temporomandibular joint, extending upward to the outer tip of the right eyebrow and backward to the right edge of the ear.
Massage: *light.*

D   Left parietal zone: area beginning 1½ finger widths to the left of the midline of the head and ending at the tip of the left ear. The front border aligns vertically with the tip of the ear and extends backward 3 finger widths.
Massage: *light.*

E   Left laterocervical zone: area ⅜ inch in diameter under the curve of the jawbone on the left side of the neck just on the median line.
Massage: *light.*

F   Right forearm zone: area ⅜ inch in diameter located on the inner right forearm 4¾ inches below the fold of the elbow.
Massage: *light.*

G   Right thigh zone: area ⅜ inch in diameter located on the front of the right thigh 2 finger widths below the horizontal line passing through the middle of the thigh and 2 finger widths to the outside of the median line.
Massage: *light.*

H   Right foot zone: long rectangular area on the top of the right foot extending from the line of the ankle to cover the first and second toes.
Massage: *light.*

I   Left foot zone: long rectangular area on the top of the left foot extending from the line of the ankle to cover the third and fourth toes.
Massage: *light.*

J   Left shoulder zone: rectangular area on the back of the left shoulder to the outside of the median clavicular line.
Massage: *light.*

K   Left buttock zone: area high on the outer side of the left buttock, located on the median axial line and on the horizontal line passing through the middle of the buttock.
Massage: *light.*

L   Lumbosacral zone: extends 1½ inches to the left and right of the line of the lower spinal vertebrae.
Massage: *light.*

M   Right palm zone: area covering the thumb and index finger and extending up the right palm to the fold of the wrist.
Massage: *light.*

N   Left hand zone: area covering the little and ring fingers and half of the middle finger and extending down the back of the left hand to the fold of the wrist.
Massage: *light.*

O   Right leg zone: rectangular area located on the back of the right lower leg from the median line of the leg to the middle of the calf, 2 finger widths below the fold of the right knee.
Massage: *light.*

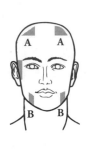

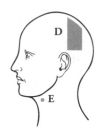

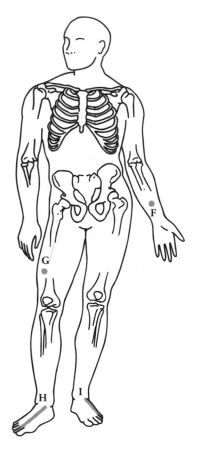

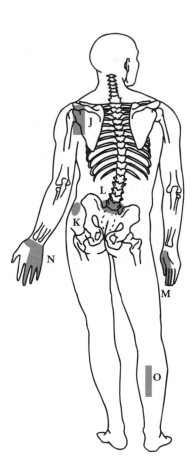

HOLLY

16
Honeysuckle
Lonicera caprifolium

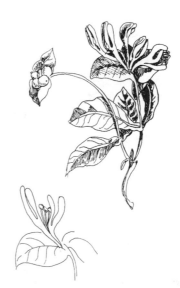

Family: Caprifoliaceae

Habitat: Europe, in thickets and hedges from low to middle altitudes.

Description: Woody shrub with flexible, branching, twining stalks that wind around any available support; new growth is hairy. The leaves are deciduous, opposite (2 to 2), oval to oblong, somewhat leathery, dark green on the right side, and a paler yellow green on the underside. Leaves on sterile branches are stemmed, those on fertile branches are very short-stemmed, while the middle leaves are sessile and those on top are fused 2 to 2, forming a single leaf pierced through its center by the stalk. The flowers, 1 to 1½ inches long, are borne in bunches in the center of the upper leaves and have long tubular corollas that can be either pink to light purple or yellowish white. The widened upper part of the corolla is bilabiate: the upper lip has 4 short lobes, while the lower lip is entire. There are 5 protruding stamens. Honeysuckle flowers from April through July.

Qualities:

> ❧ Capacity to live in the present moment
> ❧ Ability to learn from past mistakes
> ❧ Freedom in life from the bonds of the past

- Transformation
- Maturity
- Communion
- Inner softness
- Ability to relinquish what has been much beloved

Indicated for: those who are physically alive in the present but spiritually stuck in the past, so that they lack inner flexibility. There is a refusal on the part of the physical self to be guided by the spirit toward new development, so that it remains anchored in the past and lives in melancholy, regret, and nostalgia. People who respond to Honeysuckle dream of past events with their eyes open, absorbed by memories of things they have experienced. Out of touch with time, they seem prehistoric beings hurled forcefully into the future, while their modes of feeling and living remain antiquated. They lack the courage to abandon the burden of *was* for *is* because they fear new experiences. They collect everything they find on the street and never throw anything away, so that their homes are filled with dusty and useless old objects.

Honeysuckle adults refuse to grow; even their voices are childlike and their behaviors infantile. Children in need of this flower are helpless and fragile. In school they become homesick and lonely for their parents and frequently cry, and when they go to bed they must fall asleep clutching the blankie they had when they were one. New games and lessons are difficult for them. As adults they will be deeply conservative.

The treasures of the past transform into light and illumine the present.
My spirit lives in the physical present.
I am self-aware in the present, conscious of the flow of time.

Skin Zones of Honeysuckle

A   Thoracic zone: L-shaped area whose lower edge runs along the horizontal line passing through the xiphoid process to the point where it intersects with the median line of the left and right clavicle. On the left side of the chest it extends upward to form a second rectangle located between the third and seventh intercostal space.
Massage: *light.*

B   Right abdominal zone: triangular area extending diagonally from the tenth rib to the navel, outward along the ridge of the floating ribs, then downward from the outer edge of the ribs to the level of the navel. The apex of the triangle is at the top.
Massage: *light.*

C   Left arm zone: area ⅜ inch in diameter located 2 finger widths above the inner fold of the left elbow and 2 finger widths to the inside of the median line of the arm.
Massage: *light.*

D   Right leg zone: rectangular area on the front of the lower right leg, beginning 2 finger widths below the kneecap and extending downward about 3½ inches.
Massage: *light.*

E   Right dorsal zone: area ⅜ inch in diameter located along the median posterior clavicular line on the right side of the back, 2 finger widths above the lower edge of the rib cage.
Massage: *light.*

F   Left thigh zone: area ⅜ inch in diameter, located at the border between the upper and middle thirds of the leg on the back of the left thigh, 1 finger width behind the lateral line of the body.
Massage: *light.*

G   Left popliteal zone: area 1 inch in diameter in the center of the popliteal cave at the back of the left knee.
Massage: *light.*

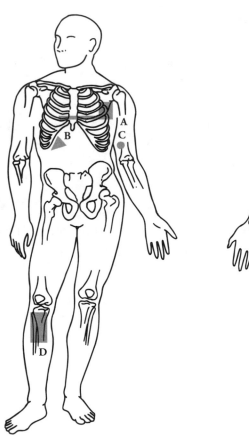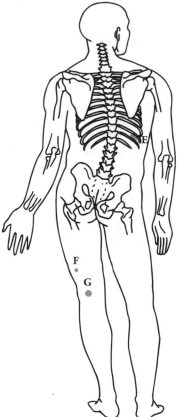

HONEYSUCKLE

17
Hornbeam
Carpinus betulus (European Hornbeam)

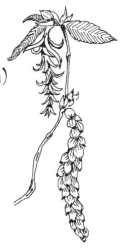

Family: Corylaceae

Habitat: Humid woods of plains, hills, and mountains up to 3,200 feet throughout Europe. Principally associated with beech and oak, it prefers very deep and loosely packed soils.

Description: Tree that may reach 80 feet in height, having a dense crown and straight trunk. The bark is smooth and ash gray, very similar to beech bark. The leaves are alternate, distichous, oblong, and simple, up to 2 feet long and 1 to 2 inches wide in size, and doubly serrated at the edges, dark green on top and an opaque light green on the bottom. The monoecious flowers are carried in catkins. The male flowers are cylindrical, ¾ to 1½ inches long, without bracts, and have broad, dark red scales. The female flowers are shorter, with 3 scales to each node. The fruit-bearing bracts are composed of 3 lobes, the middle lobe being 2 to 3 times as long as the lateral lobes. Hornbeam flowers from March through May.

Qualities:

- Vitality
- Strength and energy
- Inner vivacity
- Renewal of spiritual qualities
- Stress reduction

- Mental clarity
- Mental energy
- Motivation
- Diminuition of procrastination
- Strength to carry out personal intentions

Indicated for: persons who are perpetually tired and unmotivated and who wake up each morning already exhausted. Monday morning becomes a nightmare of suffering for such individuals, who remain in bed until the last moment under the illusion that time will stop. They are afraid to make any important decisions, and tasks and events loom up before them like towering and insurmountable mountains. Since the willpower is apparently exhausted and the mind has lost its vividness and elasticity, each day runs along an automatic track.

This remedy is useful for people who overuse their minds to the point of exhaustion, or paralyze them through excessive recourse to TV or computer games.

Hornbeam children come into class dragging their backpacks, shuffling their feet along the floor as if they don't have the strength to lift them. Seated at their desks, they instantly slip into a slouch, and while their friends are out playing at recess, they remain seated or lie down in some corner with a headache. They have the feeling that their bodies are totally devoid of energy because there is no energetic flow between mind and body. For this reason they crave all kinds of stimulants in order to simply make it through the day until evening finally comes.

I perceive inner strength as an ocean of energy.
I have the willpower to initiate projects and bring them to conclusion.
I reintegrate my skills and abilities, bringing them into the present.

Skin Zones of Hornbeam

A Upper right arm zone: area ⅜ inch in diameter, located on the front of the upper right arm between the median and external lateral lines of the body, 2 finger widths below the armpit.
Massage: *light.*

B Right thoracic zone: area about 3 inches in diameter on the median axial line, 3 finger widths below the fold of the armpit on the right side of the chest.
Massage: *light.*

C Right arm zone: long rectangular area on the inner side of the right arm, covering the lower third of the upper arm and the higher third of the forearm.
Massage: *light.*

D Bilateral femoral zone: area 1 inch in diameter located on the lateral line at the level of the top of the femur on both the left and right sides of the body.
Massage: *light.*

E Right shoulder zone: area ⅜ inch in diameter located on the back of the right shoulder, ⅜ inch to the inside of the median clavicular line and ⅜ inch above the scapular spine.
Massage: *light.*

F Left hip zone: rectangular area located high on the left hip, extending from the iliac crest upward to the ninth rib on the median axial line of the body.
Massage: *light.*

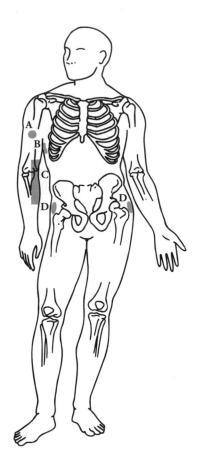
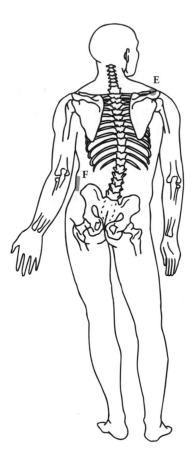

HORNBEAM

18

Impatiens

Impatiens glandulifera

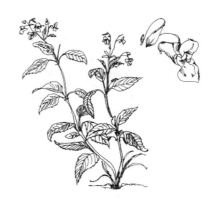

Family: Balsaminaceae

Habitat: Originally native to the Himalayas, impatiens is becoming rapidly widespread in Europe, especially in humid, marshy, or boggy environments.

Description: Plant varying in height from 3 to 5 feet having thick, spreading, succulent branches and a strongly disagreeable odor. The ovate leaves are light green. The pink flowers are 2 inches long, with two lips and a thick, narrow, pointed spur folded underneath them, and are arranged in terminal and axillary panicles. Impatiens flowers from June through September.

Qualities:

- Patience
- Spontaneity
- Relaxation
- Acceptance of what *is*
- Tolerance
- Recognition of other people's rhythms
- Freedom from tension

Indicated for: those whose interior rhythm is so fast-paced that they are afraid they will not be able to stay tuned in to it. The outer world moves much more slowly than they do, leaving them feeling like the motor of a souped-up sports car in the chassis of an old '40s Ford. Their brains think quickly, without respite; they are working even at night. The physical self, in trying to keep up with this incessant rhythm, becomes frenetic, always in movement, capable of carrying out a hundred tasks at once. Impatiens people can be talking on the telephone, dictating the day's agenda to their secretary, and writing a speech all at the same time.

They are in a constant state of anticipation and urge everyone around them to do as they do, instantly attacking each task and accomplishing it in a rush. Such people are unable to sit still in their chairs and are perpetually moving their arms or legs. They are apt to develop nervous tics in their cheeks or lower eyelids. Living in a kind of internal frenzy, they are often lonely since their intolerance of other people's rhythms isolates them.

Even as small children Impatiens individuals cannot manage to sit still; they are continually climbing in and out of bed at night, and will ride their bikes, for instance, with maniacal velocity. Because they are in such a rush this type of child is always tripping over things, falling down, and breaking things. In school such children fume with impatience if the teacher repeats an explanation to help a slower classmate, and are always first to raise a hand with answers to questions.

_____

I feel and am receptive to the rhythm of the world.
I am calm and serene within myself.
I accept the pace of others with patience.

_____

Skin Zones of Impatiens

A   Head zone: rectangular zone on the top of the head beginning 3 finger widths above the hairline on a line that extends from the

tips of both ears. The zone extends 1½ finger widths to the right and left of the midline of the head.
Massage: *light.*

B   Left frontal zone: area ⅜ inch in diameter on the left side of the forehead, about midway between the hairline and the left eyebrow.
Massage: *strong.*

C   Left eyebrow zone: extends from the inner third of the left eyebrow to its outer tip.
Massage: *light.*

D   Right thoracic zone: area located on the parasternal line in the fourth intercostal space on the right side of the chest.
Massage: *light.*

E   Left palm zone: area ⅜ inch in diameter in the center of the hypothenar eminence, on the interdigital line of the left thumb.
Massage: *light.*

F   Right dorsal zone: area ⅜ inch in diameter located 2 finger widths from the median clavicular line and horizontally aligned with the middle of the upper arm.
Massage: *strong.*

G   Lumbosacral zone: extends 1½ inches to the right and the left of the line of the lower spinal vertebrae.
Massage: *light.*

H   Left forearm zone: rectangular area beginning at the tip of the left elbow and extending 7 finger widths down the forearm. One side margin aligns vertically with the outer edge of the little finger, the other with the ridge of the ulna.
Massage: *light.*

I   Left popliteal zone: area 1 inch in diameter located in the center of the popliteal cave at the back of the left knee.
Massage: *light.*

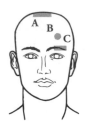

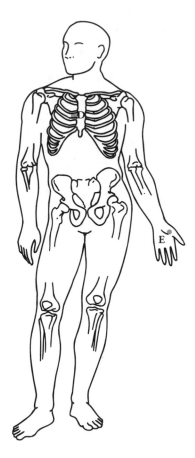

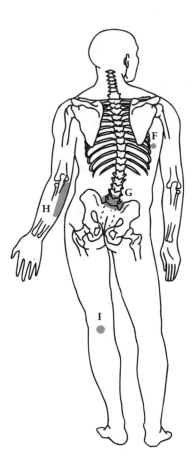

IMPATIENS

19
Larch
Larix decidua (European Larch)

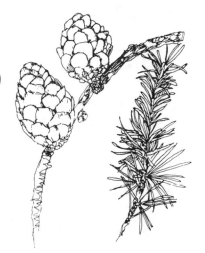

Family: Pinaceae

Habitat: In the mountains of central Europe and the Alps, where it grows spontaneously in pure stands or in woods mixed with pine at high altitudes reaching the upper limit of arboreal vegetation. At these very high elevations it may assume squat, contorted forms. At intermediate altitudes it is found in mixed forests with spruce, pine, and fir. At low altitudes larch is present in mixed woods with beech and hornbeam. It is closely related to the American larch, also known as tamarack.

Description: A large tree with a tall, thin, straight trunk and very rapid first growth, which may reach 130 feet in height and 5 feet in diameter. Larch is the only deciduous conifer in Europe. The crown is sparse and light, composed of whorled branches and smaller, pendulous branchlets. The leaves are herbaceous needles 1 to 1¼ inches long, grouped on their twigs in bundles or tufts. Before falling they assume a lovely golden yellow color. Male and female inflorescences are borne simultaneously on two- to three-year-old branches: the male catkins are small, short, and yellow, while the females are oval or cylindrical, about 2½ inches long, erect, red or purple—or more rarely, greenish or white—and arranged at the base of a rosette of leaves. Larch flowers in April and May, before its leaves come out.

Qualities:

- Confidence in one's own capacities
- Self-respect
- Conviction in one's own actions
- Stimulation of latent expressivity
- Courage
- Tenacity
- Perseverance

Indicated for: persons who feel incompetent even when they know they are not. Rather than embracing processes of continual change inherent in experiences, they refuse to face new situations and so their lives are impoverished. Hesitant and passive, they are masters of procrastination and live with a feeling of constant failure and the inevitability of negative results. Living according to assumptions of incapacity and resigned to being severely limited, they soon find the simplest daily tasks impossible.

Fear of failure sparks an inner feeling of having failed already. Their life force is extinguished and they are left in a dark room where no one has ever turned on the light. They move around in fear, since they neither perceive nor understand the things around them. Their center of creativity becomes a swamp of quicksand.

Children in need of Larch are without self-confidence. They feel like losers the moment they get out of bed and have trouble deciding which clothes to wear and what snack to bring for recess at school. In class they seldom volunteer answers and, when called on, they blush, stammer, and have great difficulty expressing themselves. They are unwilling to participate in the Christmas play, unwilling to carry the school standard to the game, and generally unwilling to compete with others, so that they are often afraid even to answer the phone.

Rivers of faith flow out from my inner world.
I accept challenges with boldness and courage.
I leave my limitations behind and proceed with certainty.

Skin Zones of Larch

A   Right thoracic zone: area about ⅜ inch in diameter located on the median axial line 3 finger widths below the fold of the arm-pit.
Massage: *light.*

B   Right hand zone: area located on the back of the right hand and extending from the fold of the wrist to the tips of the fingers from the median line of the third finger to the median line of the fifth finger.
Massage: *light.*

C   Left thigh zone: area about 1 inch in diameter located 4 finger widths above the kneecap on the front of the left thigh.
Massage: *light.*

D   Left knee zone: area located just above the upper edge of the left kneecap and 2 finger widths to the outside of the axial line.
Massage: *strong.*

E   Right knee zone: area 1 inch in diameter on the medial surface of the right knee, on the lateral line.
Massage: *light.*

F   Right leg zone: area ⅜ inch in diameter located on the lower right leg about 3 inches above the ankle bone and ¼ inch in front of the lateral line.
Massage: *light.*

G   Left elbow zone: area ⅜ inch in diameter on the inner left arm located 1 finger width above the fold of the elbow on the lateral line.
Massage: *light.*

H   Right forearm zone: rectangular area on the medial side of the right forearm, extending from the fold of the wrist to the middle of the forearm.
Massage: *light.*

I   Right dorsal zone: area ⅜ inch in diameter located 1 finger width to the right of the spinous processes of the vertebrae and 2 finger widths below the fold of the right armpit.
Massage: *light.*

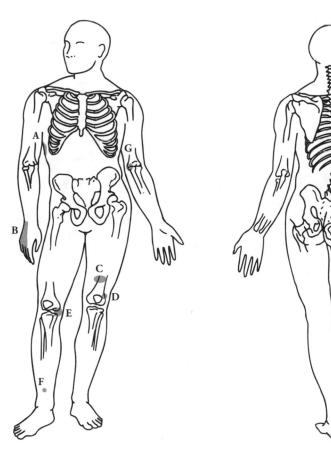

LARCH

20
Mimulus
Mimulus guttatus

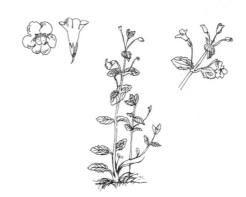

Family: Scrophulariaceae

Habitat: In North America and naturalized in Europe, having spontaneous growth and found along riverbanks and streams, and in marshes and bogs.

Description: Short-lived herbaceous plant of variable height, reaching a maximum of 2 feet. The leaves are opposite, oval, and irregularly toothed. The flowers are large, with a diameter between 1 and 1¾ inches and a flask-shaped calyx. The yellow petals are tubular and bilabiate, the lower lip being much longer than the higher lip; the throat is mottled with red. Mimulus flowers from June through September.

Qualities:

- Courage
- Trust
- Security
- Dissolution of anxiety
- Release from the phantom of fear

Indicated for: those who feel that they are constant magnets for traumatic and catastrophic events and therefore live in fear. Everything becomes a mad undertaking, even leaving the house, going shopping, driving the car, or taking the bus. Such people feel inwardly fragile, almost as if they were made of very thin glass that could break into pieces at the least vibration.

People in need of this remedy look out on the world with timidity, as if they had not yet experienced real life. They fear everything, even their own sensations, and worry about people's reactions, whether the plane will stay up, and whether or not the neighbor's dog will bite them. In fact they have very little actual experience and open themselves to the phenomenal world with an inherent wish to escape it, since their spirit has not brought past experience to consciousness. They may become hypersensitive to whatever is happening: cold, wind, noises, or smells.

Children who respond to this remedy open their eyes in the morning and instead of smiling at their mother, begin to cry. At school they are timid and apt to blush. They have a hard time parting from their mothers and do so only after much weeping and shouting. These children are startled by the slightest sound, from a pencil falling onto the floor or the neighbor blowing his nose to the shrill screech of chalk scratching the blackboard.

The universe is a safe place.
I find the courage inside myself to move toward new experiences.
I accept the manifestations of the world and open myself in the certitude of safety.

Skin Zones of Mimulus

A   Right lateral cervical zone: rectangular area ½ inch wide, beginning at the level of the tip of the right ear and ending at the base of the neck.
Massage: *light.*

B   Bilateral shoulder zone: area ¾ inch in diameter located on the front of both shoulders where they meet with the pectoral muscles. Massage: *light*.

C   Inner left arm zone: ¾-inch-wide rectangular area on the inner side of the left arm, beginning at the shoulder and extending to cover the upper third of the left forearm. Massage: *light*.

D   Left pelvic zone: area ¾ inch in diameter located on the front left side of the pelvis just above the top of the femur. Massage: *light*.

E   Left thigh zone: area 1 inch in diameter located 4 finger widths above the kneecap on the front of the left thigh. Massage: *light*.

F   Right leg zone: area ⅜ inch in diameter located on the inner front side of the lower right leg, 3 inches above the inner ankle bone and ¼ inch in front of the lateral line. Massage: *strong*.

G   Cervical zone: oval area located over the seventh cervical vertebra. Massage: *light*.

H   Spinal zone: area running down the dorsal vertebrae, beginning with the third and ending at the eighth vertebra on the line of the spinous process. Massage: *light*.

I   Lumbosacral zone: extends for 1½ inches to the left and right of the line of the lower spinal vertebrae. Massage: *light*.

J   Left elbow zone: area ⅜ inch in diameter on the inner fold of the left elbow. Massage: *strong*.

K   Area covering the entire sole of the right foot. Massage: *light*.

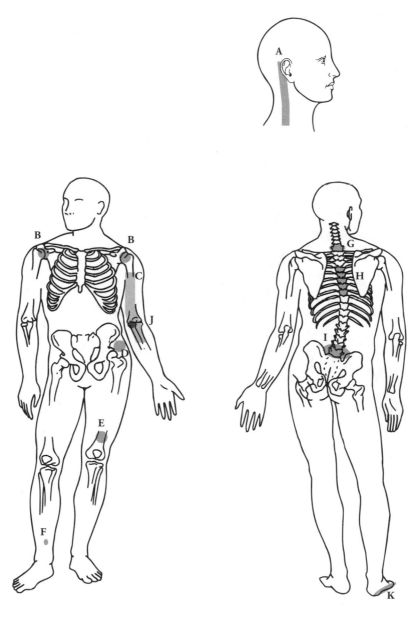

MIMULUS

21
Mustard
Sinapis arvensis

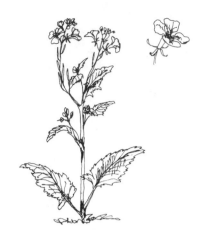

Family: Cruciferae

Habitat: Common in open fields, meadows, and uncultivated land throughout Europe.

Description: Annual plant 1 to 2 feet high, covered in light, sparse hairs. The basal leaves are stemless, pinnate, lobed, and lyre-shaped; the upper leaves are simple and almost entire and do not wrap around the stalk. The light yellow flowers have narrow sepals that widen horizontally and two stamens, and are borne in terminal bunches, opening one after the other. Mustard flowers from May to September.

Qualities:

- Joy
- Illumination of sadness
- Transcendence of melancholy
- Serenity
- Clarity in interior darkness
- Antidote to misery
- Gaiety

Indicated for: those who feel dogged by an unidentifiable dark cloud following them everywhere, at times intensifying, at times dispersing. Such people have the unconscious sensation of having lived through traumatic experiences, which have left behind obscure and bitter memories. In certain moments they perceive situations to be analogous to events they have experienced before. Their souls seem to be sad and sullen, unable to radiate the light of the spirit; in fact, they feel distant from the spirit, not fully interpenetrant. Hoping to avoid any real connection, they isolate themselves, cease to perceive the present, and fall into immobility and creative impotence. Everything, even speaking, turns into the most extreme suffering, and life seems a dream lived in the darkness, bereft of feelings and color. Finally, unable to progress, they fall into a lethargic state in which they feel hurled into a bottomless well in a terrible free-fall.

They cannot seem to link up with the positive force of the soul and so nourish their bodies with light. Theirs are souls veiled in black silk, living in the middle of darkness.

This is the fall into the earthly realm of the human being who cannot remember why it has happened, only that she or he has been ejected from the world of light to the world of shadows and suffering.

Children who respond to Mustard are always sad and morose and hardly ever produce a spontaneous smile. Introverts, they may suddenly start to cry and refuse to be consoled or otherwise lose all interest and refuse to be engaged.

Full to the brim with joy, I dance through the world.
I shine with the light and strength of the spirit.
I open my heart to divine love.

Skin Zones of Mustard

A   Neck zone: area ⅜ inch in diameter located at the base of the left side of the neck on the lateral line.
Massage: *light.*

B Right shoulder zone: area ⅜ inch in diameter located 1 finger width to the inside of the elongation of the anterior axial line and 2 finger widths below the acromion.
Massage: *strong*.

C Bilateral elbow zone: oval area on the inner fold of both the left and right arm.
Massage: *light*.

D Left thigh zone: area 1 inch in diameter just under the inguinal fold on the left side of the body.
Massage: *light*.

E Bilateral wrist zone: oval area on the inner wrist of both the left and right arms.
Massage: *light*.

F Left palm zone: area ⅜ inch in diameter located on the left palm just below the interdigital space between the axial line of the middle and ring fingers.
Massage: *strong*.

G Left thigh zone: area 1 inch in diameter located 4 finger widths above the left kneecap on the front of the thigh.
Massage: *light*.

H Right leg zone: area ⅜ inch in diameter located on the lower right leg about 3 inches above the inner ankle bone and ¼ inch in front of the lateral line.
Massage: *strong*.

I Right foot zone: area ⅜ inch in diameter located on the top of the right foot to the inside of the axial line, 2 finger widths under the articular line of the foot.
Massage: *light*.

J Right foot zone: area covering the inner side of the right foot from just under the inner ankle bone around to the back of the heel and frontward to the arch of the foot.
Massage: *light*.

K Left cheek zone: rectangular area ¾ inch high, beginning at the level of the left corner of the lips and extending upward to where the left earlobe joins to the cheek.
Massage: *light.*

L Bilateral arm zone: rectangular area located just to the inside of the median line, beginning at the fold of the elbow and extending upward to almost the midpoint of the upper arm on both the left and right arms.
Massage: *light.*

M Left dorsal zone: rectangular area 1 inch wide extending from the iliac crest upward to the tenth rib and vertically aligned with the median clavicular line on the left side of the back.
Massage: *light.*

N Left thigh zone: area 1 inch in diameter located on the median line in the middle third of the back of the left thigh.
Massage: *light.*

O Right knee zone: area ⅜ inch in diameter located 1 inch below the inner fold on the back of the right knee and 1 finger width to the outside of the axial line.
Massage: *strong.*

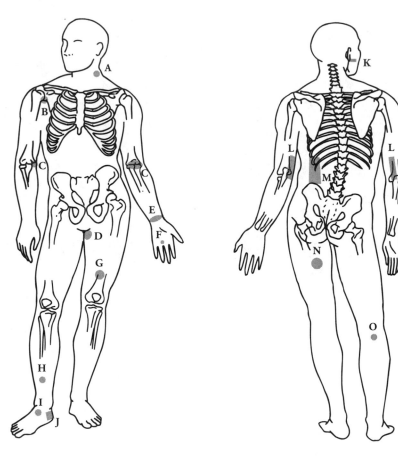

MUSTARD

22
Oak
Quercus robur (English Oak)

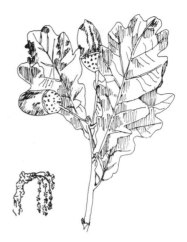

Family: Fagaceae

Habitat: Native to Europe, North Africa, and West Asia, naturalized in southeastern Canada and the northeastern United States, and planted in southeastern and Pacific states. Oak thrives in cool, rich, deep soils in pure and mixed forests of hills and mountains up to 5,800 feet in altitude.

Description: Growing up to 160 feet high and 6½ feet in diameter, English oak is one of the most characteristic of British trees and may live to be 1,000 years old. The crown is broad, open, rounded, and irregular. The leaves are asymmetrical at the base, alternate, simple, deciduous, and herbaceous. They are narrow at the base, widening toward the top, with 5 to 7 pairs of broad lobes, carried on very short stems, and are a shiny light green on the upper side. The male flowers, borne on pendulous catkins that develop from buds on the branch from the previous year, spring from a slightly hairy axis carrying about 12 flowers with greenish yellow perianths and 4 to 12 stamens with hairless anthers. The female flowers, with 3 blackish red stigmas, are arranged in spikes from 1¼ to 2 inches long, formed by a smooth, shiny axis bearing from 2 to more than 5 flowers. English oak flowers between April and June.

Qualities:

- Strength
- Tenacity

- Reliability
- Courage in the face of adversity
- Reestablishment of equilibrium through rest
- Playful flexibility in work and commitments
- Perseverance

Indicated for: those who tend to bear the weight of the world on their shoulders, becoming pillars of the community and demonstrating strength and endurance. As they are certain that their souls are great and immortal, they seldom falter or complain about the hard daily work they take on. Life, they reason, is a time of effort and struggle.

Their high ideals sustain such people, inspiring them with an almost superhuman tenacity, commitment, and capacity to take on others' responsibilities and resolve their problems.

Oak individuals are disposed to sacrifice and work and seldom make time for rest. At times they do not even realize how much they are asking of themselves and their poor bodies until they have completely worn them out, so that they are suddenly seized by physical difficulty, such as severe lower back pain, that immobilizes them. Then everything seems to come to a grinding halt, physically and psychically, and they become sad and worried about not being able to fulfill their commitments.

Children who need Oak are forever taken up with their play and study projects; their days are so crammed with appointments as to look like some corporate manager's agenda. They become absorbed in their interests to the point of exhaustion, and study till late at night or wake up early in the morning to read "those last two lines of Chapter 10 in the history book."

Energy and strength are my spiritual inheritance.
I nourish my own joy and flexibility in every undertaking.
I persevere with tenacity yet understand the desire for rest.

Skin Zones of Oak

A   Left cheekbone zone: rectangular area whose inner margin lies about 1¼ inches from the left side of the nose and whose outer margin aligns vertically with the outer corner of the left eyebrow, extending from the lower edge of the left eye socket downward to the bottom of the nose.
Massage: *light.*

B   Bilateral wrist zone: oval area on the inside of both the left and right wrists.
Massage: *light.*

C   Left palm zone: rectangular area extending from the fold of the left wrist to the tips of the outer fingers. The lateral border begins at the middle of the wrist and extends to the inside edge of the middle finger; the medial border extends along the outer edge of the left hand to the outer corner of the little finger.
Massage: *light.*

D   Bilateral ankle zone: area 1 inch in diameter located just above the inner ankle bone on the inner front side of both legs.
Massage: *light.*

E   Right foot zone: area ⅜ inch in diameter located on the lateral line of the body 1 finger width above the sole of the right foot.
Massage: *strong.*

F   Right cervical zone: rectangular area on the right side of the back of the neck extending from the horizontal line passing through the base of the right earlobe to the base of the neck, 1 finger width from the median vertebral line.
Massage: *light.*

G   Bilateral shoulder zone: area 1 inch in diameter located on the back of both the left and right shoulder on the posterior axial line (or elongation).
Massage: *light.*

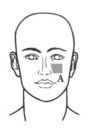

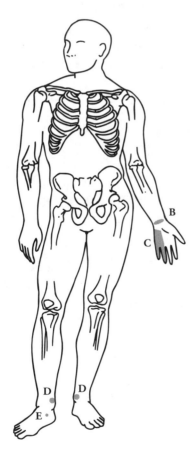

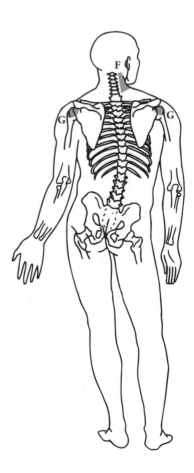

OAK

23
Olive
Olea europaea

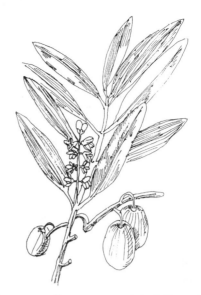

Family: Oleaceae

Habitat: Olive was probably originally native to Asia Minor, but has long been widely dispersed throughout the Mediterrenean region due to cultivation.

Description: A small evergreen tree with a spreading crown. Height, which may reach 65 feet, varies according to the age of the tree, the variety cultivated, and the environment in which it is grown. The trunk is narrow, cylindrical, and twisted, with a circumference proportionate to the age of the tree. The bark, smooth and gray in young plants, turns darker and becomes mottled and furrowed in adult trees. The rather small, silver-green leaves are ellipsoid to lanceolate with entire margins and are leathery, opposed, and covered with densely matted hairs on the underside, a characteristic that saves them from excessive water loss during the hot Mediterranean summers. The flowers are small and white, formed in dense axillary inflorescences. The corolla is composed of 4-petaled, milky white lobes; the calyx is gamosepalous, green, small, and divided into oval lobes; there are 2 stamens with protruding anthers; the ovary is superior, sessile, free, and oval with 2 lobes, each containing 2 ovules for each of the 2 loculi; the style is short and the stigma is forked. Olive flowers from March through June.

Qualities:

- Awareness of one's own limits
- Regeneration from the spiritual source
- Renewal
- Inner peace
- Recognition of self-abuse
- Tranquility
- Balance
- Vitality and strength

Indicated for: those who feel inwardly worn out, tired to the point of total exhaustion. Such people have come to the end of their rope after having made excessive demands on their physical, emotional, or mental bodies. Although they are burned out, they still do not realize that they must stop, since they neither see nor reflect on their condition. At first they alternate between phases of great productivity and times of exhaustion, but in the end their batteries run down. In this condition every form of inner life is swept away as if in a great flood. All hope of continuing on with life, of rebirth or rejuvenation, is gone, since illness has reduced them to human shadows who no longer believe in their own survival. They develop a mantra of exhaustion: "I can't make it anymore, it's all too much."

Individuals in need of Olive may be on a spiritual path, driving themselves daily to the breaking point to fulfill their spiritual ideals. When they are almost there, they suddenly give up the quest for lack of remaining strength.

Children responsive to this remedy are perpetually tired and weak and in need of recharging. They may fall ill easily then seem to get better, but two days later be back in bed with a fever.

I reconnect with the energy of the cosmos and allow it to flow through me.
I find the strength for self-regeneration within me.
I live in an unfolding process of peace.

Skin Zones of Olive

A Right frontal zone: rectangular area located on the right side of the forehead, beginning at the hairline and extending above the right eyebrow. The outside margin aligns vertically with the outside tip of the eyebrow; the inside margin lies 1½ finger widths to the side of the midline.
Massage: *light.*

B Right parasternal zone: area ⅜ inch in diameter located on the right side of the chest in the fourth intercostal space.
Massage: *light.*

C Sternal zone: area about ⅜ inch in diameter located at the level of acupuncture point CV17 on the sternum.
Massage: *light.*

D Right costal zone: area 1 inch in diameter located on the curve of the right side of the rib cage on the paravertebral line at the level of the horizontal line passing through the xiphoid process.
Massage: *light.*

E Right abdominal zone: area located below the horizontal umbilical line on the right side of the abdomen just over the iliac crest.
Massage: *light.*

F Right foot zone: area ⅜ inch in diameter located on the lateral line of the body on the inner side of the right foot, 1 finger width above the sole.
Massage: *strong.*

G Bilateral trapezoid zone: rectangular area extending 6 finger widths to the left and right of the spine, beginning at the level of the sixth cervical vertebra at the upper edge of the trapezius muscle and ending at the level of the second thoracic vertebra.
Massage: *light.*

H Lumbar zone: area located at the level of the first lumbar vertebra on the median vertebral line.
Massage: *light.*

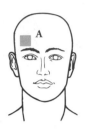

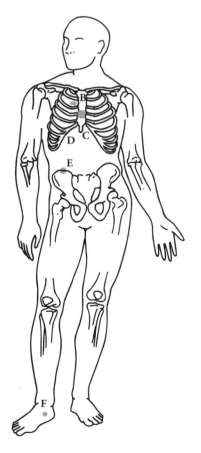

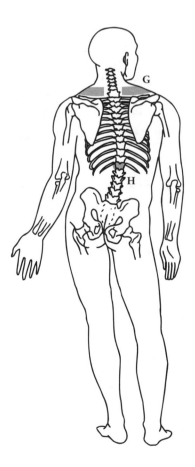

OLIVE

24
Pine
Pinus sylvestris (Scotch Pine)

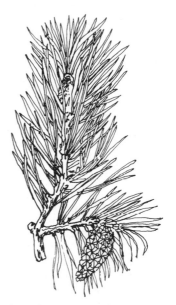

Family: Pinaceae

Habitat: Native to the Scottish Highlands and spontaneous throughout Europe and northern Asia south to Turkey, naturalized in southeastern Canada and in the northeastern United States from New England west to Iowa. Commercially grown as shelterbelts, Christmas trees, and ornamentals, Scotch Pine is the most widely distributed pine in the world and thrives in a variety of soils from loamy to sandy.

Description: Easily distinguishable from other pines by its orange-red bark, which forms scaly plates on the upper part of the trunk and branches. Its foliage is a rich blue green and is composed of flexible, twisting, 1½- to 3-inch-long needles grouped in pairs or, more rarely, in bundles of 3 to 5. These needles are persistent for about 3 years. The crown is pointed in young trees, flattened in older trees. Scotch Pine is a monoecious plant bearing sporophylls in 3-inch-long, oblong to ovate, reddish yellow catkins around continuously growing new shoots. The ovoid macrosporophylls, 4 inches long, solitary, and reflexive, are carried just under the apical bud and are almost spherical with a fairly long peduncle. The sporophylls open from May through June.

Qualities:

> ⚘ Dissolution of guilt
> ⚘ Forgiveness

- Compassion
- Repentance
- Acceptance
- Relinquishment of remorse
- Assumption of responsibility in appropriate measure
- Comprehension of error as life's greatest teacher
- Redemption

Indicated for: those who feel a sense of guilt ranging from original sin to having forgotten to telephone an acquaintance. They are always asking pardon or saying, "I'm sorry . . . excuse me . . . I didn't mean to." They view their souls as stained for having done something, although they cannot remember what it was, and go through life with this flaw continually coloring each event of their existence. They beat their breasts and cry, "Mea culpa, mea culpa, mea massima culpa," without perceiving that it is human to err and that we must learn from every mistake in order not to repeat it.

Immersed in guilt, Pine people punish themselves, bearing their crosses alone. They feel inferior and unhappy, subservient to a destiny that casts the blame on them. They may not even believe they deserve to live on this earth and often feel they have failed to meet their parents' expectations. Their bodies are not illumined by the joy of life, since they always have the sensation of having done something wrong, even if it is only eating a chocolate late at night when no one is looking. They tire quickly and severely, exhausting themselves, and their vitality is extinguished in the shadow of the struggle between right and wrong and good and evil.

Children who need Pine feel that their parents are always admonishing them, acusing them of having done something or other. At school they take the blame for crimes committed by their companions, or by their brother or sister. They become innocent victims of society and, if unjustly accused, they do not defend themselves but masochistically accept their punishment.

❧❧❧

I live in divine forgiveness, for the redemption of my soul.
I accept my mistakes as expressions of life on the spiritual path.
I dissolve my sense of guilt with the light of love.

❧❧❧

SKIN ZONES OF PINE

A   Upper left jaw zone: 2-inch-wide rectangular area located at the level of the temporomandibular articulation of the jaw in front of the left ear, extending from the base of the earlobe upward to the beginning of the hairline.
Massage: *light.*

B   Lower left jaw zone: rectangle beginning horizontal to the left corner of the mouth and ending at the lower ridge of the jaw-bone. The front margin aligns vertically with the outside tip of the left eyebrow and the zone extends backward toward the ear till it meets the jaw.
Massage: *light.*

C   Head zone: long rectangular area running down the back of the head, beginning 3 finger widths behind the crown and ending at the occipital ridge. It extends 1½ finger widths to both the left and right of the head's midline.
Massage: *light.*

D   Right shoulder zone: area covering the whole of the right shoulder, back and front, from its articulation down to the upper third of the right arm on the internal and external axial lines at the level of the armpit.
Massage: *light.*

E   Bilateral subclavicular zone: area ¾ inch in diameter located just below the outer, lower ridge of the clavicle on both the left and

right sides of the body.
Massage: *light.*

F   Epigastric zone: area bordered on both sides by the costal arch and covering the xiphoid process. This zone varies in height, depending on the individual's constitution and thoracic configuration.
Massage: *light.*

G   Bilateral femoral zone: area 1 inch in diameter located on the lateral line of the body at the level of the top of both the left and right femurs.
Massage: *light.*

H   Right pelvic zone: area 1 inch in diameter located to the right of the median line just above the pubic tubercle.
Massage: *light.*

I   Right thigh zone: 1½-inch-wide rectangle on the front of the right thigh, extending from a horizontal line just above the kneecap upward to the upper third of the thigh. The inner border aligns vertically with the outer edge of the right kneecap.
Massage: *light.*

J   Posterior left leg zone: rectangular area on the back and outer side of the lower left leg whose inner border lies on the median posterior line and whose upper border is just above the popliteal cave at the back of the left knee. The zone extends downward to the middle of the calf.
Massage: *light.*

K   Anterior left leg zone: area ⅜ inch in diameter located about 4 inches above the bend of the ankle and 1 finger width in front of the lateral line on the left leg.
Massage: *light.*

L   Right foot zone: area ⅜ inch in diameter located on the top of the right foot just inside the axial line and 2 finger widths below the bend of the ankle.
Massage: *light.*

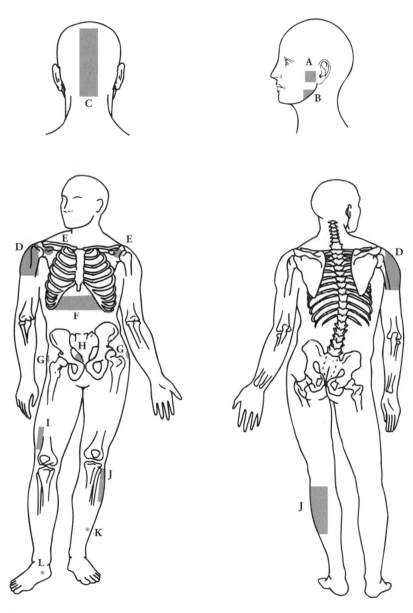

PINE

25
Red Chestnut
Aesculus carnea

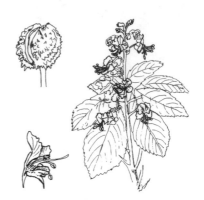

Family: Hippocastanaceae

Habitat: A hardy, drought-tolerant plant derived from the hybridization of horsechestnut and red buckeye, red chestnut is cultivated throughout Europe as a shade tree along roadways and in parks and gardens.

Description: A tree that may reach 80 feet in height, having a dense, regular crown and dark red bark. Its dark green leaves are deciduous, sometimes curled, composed of 5 almost sessile leaflets that are cuneiform and obovate with crenellated margins. The flowers consist of a rather short calyx and clavate, fringed petals varying from a light to deep pink and are borne in dense panicles up to 8 inches high. Red chestnut flowers from April through May.

Qualities:

- Devotion
- Service
- Neighborly help
- Supportive love
- Nourishment and support of others
- Healing through positive thought
- Transmission of spiritual aid
- Profound connection with oneself
- Relinquishment of overprotection for harmonious participation

Indicated for: people who live through others' lives, forgetting their own. They project their own fears on others and are incapable of cutting the umbilical with their creations, whether physical or mental. Such individuals cannot seem to let their offspring grow up on their own and fuss over them as if they were newborn, even after many years. They also do this with principles and concepts formulated long ago and now anachronistic and out of place. Apprehensive and timorous, they have never truly wanted to wean their children and allow them to go on to experience life on their own. They are unable to relinquish their hold on a family member who has married or left home, or who is about to die. The resultant inner suffering manifests as overprotectiveness and a disproportionate alarmism.

Red Chestnut people live their lives as a process of abandonment, as if their spirit, suffering through the passage into incarnation, had abandoned its primordial condition. They experience inner disconnection as suffering unaccompanied by maturation and they project it onto others in the guise of obsessive love.

As children they are apprehensive about everything, worrying about what could have happened to a friend who is absent from school, firmly believing that tomorrow will bring a catastrophe. They get sick at the drop of a hat, even if they are taking dozens of preventative medicines and wear a hat pulled down to and a scarf pulled up to their eyes. Such children may have suffered a prenatal trauma or traumatic birth experience.

I radiate divine healing light from my soul.
I nourish my body and soul with celestial love, so that I may
grow with others.
I help my fellow beings with appropriate detachment, while
inspiring them with supportive love.

Skin Zones of Red Chestnut

A Bilateral subclavicular zone: area ¾ inch in diameter located under the outer lower edge of the left and right collarbones.
   Massage: *light*.

B Right parasternal zone: area ⅜ inch in diameter on the right side of the chest on the level of the fourth intercostal space.
   Massage: *light*.

C Right hand zone: area on the back of the right hand covering the thumb and half of the index finger, ending on its axial line. The zone extends from the tips of the thumb and finger to the fold of the wrist.
   Massage: *light*.

D Right earlobe zone: area 2½ inches in diameter located on the external face of the right earlobe.
   Massage: *strong*.

E Left shoulder zone: 3½-inch-high area on the back of the left shoulder beginning at the median clavicular line and extending outward for 2 inches.
   Massage: *light*.

F Left dorsal zone: area on the left side of the back extending from the median horizontal line of the scapula to the tenth rib. Vertically it extends from the fold of the armpit to 2 finger widths to the left of the spine.
   Massage: *light*.

G Bilateral arm zone: rectangular area located to the inside of the median line of both the left and right arm, beginning at the bend of the elbow and extending upward to the middle of the upper arm.
   Massage: *light*.

H Lumbosacral zone: extends for about 1½ inches to the left and right of the line of the lower spinal vertebrae.
   Massage: *light*.

I Right posterior leg zone: area 1 inch in diameter on the back of the right lower leg above the Achilles' heel.
   Massage: *light*.

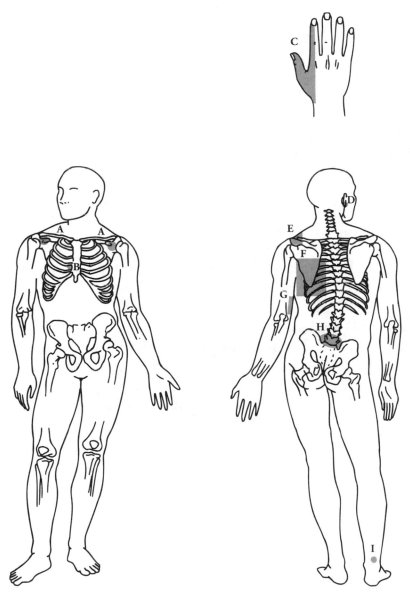

RED CHESTNUT

26
Rock Rose
Helianthemum nummularium

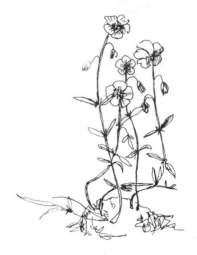

Family: Cistaceae

Habitat: Native to North America and the Mediterranean region of Europe, rock rose thrives in rocky and grassy soils, in clearings, and in limestone from low altitudes up to 5,800 feet.

Description: A shrublike plant varying in height from 4 to 6 inches and having a diameter of 2 feet, prostrate and not very woody, with branches that frequently put out roots. Its leaves, 2 to 8 inches long, vary in color from green to gray green and are densely hairy and elliptical in shape, with rounded edges on the bottom. Each leaf bears a pair of long stipules where it branches off from the leafstalk.

The flowers are composed of a visibly veined calix and 5 petals, usually yellow (rarely white or with shadings of orange or pink) and are about 8 inches in diameter, solitary, and unilateral in inflorescence. The sepals are a dense furry gray. Rock rose flowers from May through August.

Qualities:

- Transcendence of one's own small world
- Courage in confrontation with life's extreme challenges
- Harmony
- Integration
- Connection with the energies of nature

- Perseverance and bravery
- Dissolution of the sensations of terror and panic
- Freedom to move through paralyzing situations
- Tranquility and inner peace

Indicated for: those who, when faced with difficulties, perceive that they are not integrated, that the soul is unable to synchronize the spirit with the body. The spirit is seen as detached from the physical being, and the individual panics. Unable to listen to the advice of others, she can no longer see or manage to speak, but remains paralyzed, with no visible way out of her predicament.

Children who respond to this remedy are incapable of coping with crises. If they are present, for instance, when another child suffers an epileptic seizure, they will be literally unable to move and remain rooted to the spot without calling for help. They may contract a sudden, severe stomachache and vomit, remaining immobile and dazed for hours afterward.

Rock Rose is indicated for people who easily fall prey to fears induced by outward agents, for children panicked by TV coverage of a flood, for example, or for students who freeze during oral exams and go dumb or are seized by panic during class essays and cannot write a word.

This is also the remedy of choice for persons suffering from specific and extreme trauma: a natural catastrophe such as flood or earthquake, an accident, or news of terminal illness in a loved one. It is useful for those having trouble returning to the body after general anaesthesia, for people in coma, and for individuals who remain disoriented following surgery.

My spirit is integrated in harmony with my physical body.
The energy of nature flows peacefully through me.
I am able to move when confronted with paralyzing situations.

Skin Zones of Rock Rose

A   Bilateral subclavicular zone: area about ¾ inch in diameter located under the outer lower ridge of both the left and right collarbones.
Massage: *light* on the left, *strong* on the right.

B   Left abdominal zone: 1½-inch-high rectangular area located on the horizontal line passing through the navel and extending from the linea alba to the median axillary line on the left side of the abdomen.
Massage: *light.*

C   Right hip zone: area 1 inch in diameter located over the right hip joint on the horizontal line passing above the pubis.
Massage: *light.*

D   Bilateral wrist zone: oval area located just below the fold of the wrist on the left and the right arms.
Massage: *light.*

E   Lower right leg zone: rectangular area located on the inside front of the lower right leg, beginning 4 finger widths above the upper corner of the inside ankle bone and extending 6 finger widths upward and around the shin to end 5 finger widths past the midline.
Massage: *light.*

F   Right foot zone: area ⅜ inch in diameter on the top of the right foot, located 2 finger widths below the bend of the ankle to the inside of the axial line.
Massage: *light.*

G   Bilateral arm zone: rectangular area on the inside back of both upper arms, beginning at the bend of the elbow and extending upward to almost halfway up the upper arm.
Massage: *light.*

H   Left thigh zone: 2-inch-wide rectangular area on the back of the left thigh extending from the fold of the buttock to the popliteal,

to the inside of the median posterior line.
Massage: *light.*

I   Right thigh zone: 2-inch-wide rectangular area on the back of the right thigh extending from the fold of the buttock to the popliteal, 2 finger widths behind the median line of the medial face of the thigh.
Massage: *light.*

J   Right palm zone: area ⅜ inch in diameter located on the right palm 1 finger width from the axial line of the hand and the fold of the wrist.
Massage: *strong.*

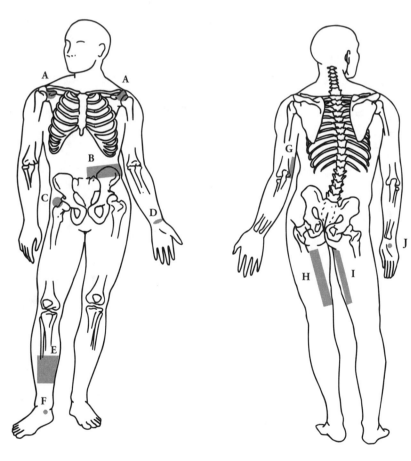

ROCK ROSE

27
Rock Water

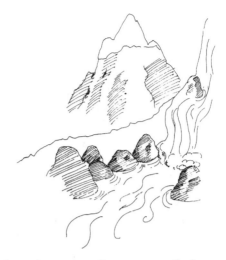

Description: This is not a plant, but water from untouched natural springs.

Qualities:

- Inner freedom
- Adaptability
- Dissolution of inner dogmatism
- Upsurge of free and open idealism
- Flexibility
- Moderation of discipline
- Elasticity
- Balance
- Renewal of playfulness
- Malleability
- Complete openness
- Creativity

Indicated for: people who are full of very high moral, social, and physical ideals and who live strictly according to those models of belief and behavior that they have constructed, succumbing to a process of rigidity and crystalization. Such individuals suffer from a sensation of having failed to respect the rules of the divine will. They feel inwardly guilty for having betrayed the trust of the Creator and so impose on themselves extreme obedience. Intransigent with themselves, ascetic and austere, they are never satisfied with what they do.

Rock Water people believe that all this will result in a more rapid evolution; they feel superior to everyone else and put themselves on pedestals—perfect statues in deserted squares. In such cases the personality desires changes that do not reflect the way the self is truly feeling. The mind, therefore, seeks to construct a kind of castle to support the personality, and dogmatic rules are the bricks of the castle's foundation.

Rock Water people fail to realize that by acting as they do they lose the dynamic forces of inner development. They may live for twenty years in an Indian or Tibetan monastery, observing all the rules, engaging in vigils, rituals, and exercises, and meditating on mantras. Then one day a toddler comes by and knocks over the platform on which they have, for the past twenty days, been constructing a perfect mandala, and chaos breaks loose. They explode in a violent and prolonged reaction of angry reproach—so much for all that hard work on holy restraint!

Children and teachers who respond to this remedy want to color the figures they are drawing without ever going outside the lines, which they feel they must respect at all costs. Rock Water infants at only two are already asking their mothers to put their toys away in precisely the right place, and if their teddy bear is in the wrong position, they get angry and cry.

I flow with the rhythm of life,
relinquishing preconstructed schemes.
I dissolve perfectionism through inner elasticity.
I break the crystals of perfection
I have so carefully constructed.

SKIN ZONES OF ROCK WATER

A   Right eyebrow zone: rectangular area covering the entire right eyebrow.
Massage: *light.*

B   Left cheek zone: area ⅜ inch in diameter located 1 finger width under and to the left of the outer corner of the left eye.
Massage: *light.*

C   Left temporal zone: rectangular area 1 inch in height on the left side of the face, extending from the upper point of attachment of the left ear to the outer corner of the left eyebrow.
Massage: *light.*

D   Left pelvic zone: 2-inch-high rectangular area beginning 1 finger width above the upper pubic bone and extending to its lower edge. It extends from the midline across the left side of the pelvis, vertically aligned on the lateral side with the back axial fold.
Massage: *light.*

E   Right knee zone: area covering the right kneecap and wrapping around the knee to cover the popliteal cave.
Massage: *light.*

F   Cervical zone: median oval area located at the level of the seventh cervical vertebra.
Massage: *strong.*

G   Right posterior shoulder zone: area ⅜ inch in diameter located on the back of the right shoulder ⅜ inch to the inside of the midpoint of the collarbone and above the spine of the scapula.
Massage: *light.*

H   Bilateral posterior shoulder zone: area about 1 inch in diameter on the posterior axillary line on the back of both the left and right shoulders.
Massage: *light.*

I   Bilateral arm zone: rectangular area on both the left and right arms located to the inside of the median axial line, beginning from the bend of the elbow and extending upward to almost the midpoint of the upper arm.
Massage: *light*.

J   Right dorsal zone: area ⅜ inch in diameter located 4 finger widths below the scapula and 2 finger widths from the median vertebral line.
Massage: *strong*.

K   Lumbosacral zone: extends for about 1½ inches to the left and right of the line of the lower spinal vertebrae.
Massage: *light*.

L   Left hand zone: area ⅜ inch in diameter on the back of the left hand, located on the trajectory of the fourth interdigital line and halfway between the interdigital space and the fold of the wrist.
Massage: *strong*.

M   Left leg zone: area ⅜ inch in diameter about 4 inches below the fold of the left knee and ⅜ inch behind the internal lateral line of the leg.
Massage: *light*.

N   Right leg zone: area 1 inch in diameter above the Achilles' heel on the back of the lower right leg.
Massage: *light*.

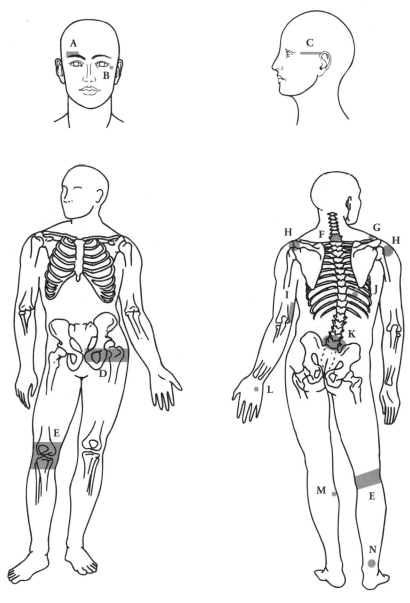

ROCK WATER

28
Scleranthus
Scleranthus annuus

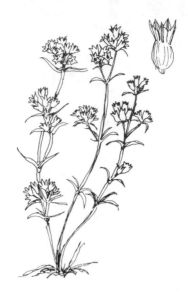

Family: Caryophyllaceae

Habitat: Native to Europe and naturalized in North America along the Pacific Coast and along the Atlantic Coast to Manitoba and Minnesota. Scleranthus thrives in arid, sandy, limeless soils from the plains to extremely high altitudes.

Description: A low-branching perennial, erect or diffuse, with short linear opposite leaves varying from 2 to 6 inches in length. The green flowers are composed of 5 united sepals without petals forming in dense clusters at the tips of the branches. Scleranthus flowers from May to October.

Qualities:

- Clarity
- Synthesis between thought and action
- Swift adaptability
- Inner stability
- Swift and correct decision making
- Security
- Concentration

Indicated for: persons who feel themselves to be without center and oscillate inwardly from one pole to the other, seeking a precarious balance. They feel enveloped by a whirlwind, by such a flood of emotions and situations that every decision soon seems the wrong one, so they accept any circumstance that happens to present itself. To the outsider it all looks very muddled and confused.

Indeed, these people lack inner clarity, stability, and balance, swinging between dual poles because the soul is unable to give them direction and measure. The spirit wants one thing, the body another; neither accepts the other with love and respect. They exist separately within reality, unwilling to communicate and interlock. The self then lives in a state of destructive duality and alienation.

A young man in need of Scleranthus may want to go for a hike in the mountains with his sweetheart on Sunday. They decide to do it on Friday, but Saturday morning he calls her to say, "I can't come, I have to do homework for Monday." That afternoon he calls back, all enthused, and says, "Look, let's go after all. It'll be a lot of fun." But Saturday evening the telephone rings: "I guess I won't be able to come, since Claudio can't come either."

The psyches of such people are riding a seesaw of emotion, always swinging between tears and laughter, love and hatred, serenity and rage. They lose a lot of opportunities since, although they want to, they can't quite manage to make personal decisions and opportunities slip through their fingers. As children they are perpetually uncertain and insecure, losing two hours at the toy store trying to decide what to buy.

Scleranthus people may be so unstable on their feet as to stagger; they are frequently dizzy and are apt to get very carsick.

I see what I must do with extreme clarity.
I feel the inward communion of body and spirit.
I am coherent and decisive.

Skin Zones of Scleranthus

A Left frontal zone: rectangular area beginning at the left side of the hairline and ending just above the left eyebrow. The outside margin aligns vertically with the outer tip of the eyebrow; the inner margin lies 1½ finger widths to the left side of the midline of the face.
Massage: *light.*

B Right thoracic zone: area ⅜ inch in diameter, located on the median axillary line 3 finger widths below the fold of the armpit on the right side of the chest.
Massage: *light.*

C Bilateral femoral zone: area 1 inch in diameter located on the median lateral line at the level of the top of the femur on both sides of the body.
Massage: *light.*

D Left thigh zone: area 1 inch in diameter located 4 finger widths above the left kneecap.
Massage: *light.*

E Left knee zone: area ⅜ inch in diameter located on the upper edge of the left kneecap, 2 finger widths from the axial line of the leg.
Massage: *strong.*

F Left leg zone: area ⅜ inch in diameter located 1 finger width in front of the lateral line of the left leg and 4 inches above the fold of the ankle.
Massage: *light.*

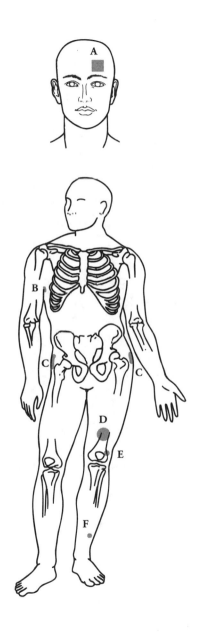

SCLERANTHUS

29
Star of Bethlehem
Ornithogalum umbellatum

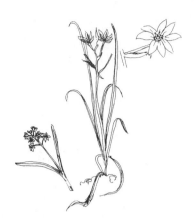

Family: Liliaceae

Habitat: Common in uncultivated fields and along roadsides throughout Europe and in North America from Newfoundland south to North Carolina.

Description: Herbaceous plant with inflorescence in broad, flat clusters formed of 15 flowers that open to the sun. The leaves can be as long as 6 inches and as wide as 2 inches and have a white stripe running down the center. The clear white flower is star-shaped with narrow sepals and is borne on a 5- to 12-inch-long stalk; the lower floral peduncles are longer than the upper ones. Star of Bethlehem flowers between April and June.

Qualities:

- Freedom from traumatic influences originating in the past
- Reorientation after shock
- Reawakening
- Peace and serenity in the midst of chaos
- Rebirth
- Inner vitality
- Inner healing
- Dissolution of pain linked to physical and psychic traumas

Indicated for: people who feel blocked in their expression and uneasy in certain situations without knowing why. Whether or not they are aware of it, a past trauma is still alive in them, manifesting itself in emotional and physical paralysis and causing aches and pains in the muscles and joints. Certain parts of the body refuse to work properly and throw off the whole system. Then these individuals feel off balance, as though without a hand, shoulder, or knee. Suffering from an energetic block that prohibits the harmonious flow of energy throughout the body, they feel anaesthetized in certain areas.

All the traumas of life—from birth and weaning to surgery, car accidents, miscarriage, divorce, dismissal, and the first day of school—can be eased by use of this remedy.

Children in need of it go to school every day complaining of stomach- or headaches. Their incomprehensible behavior may be the result of something that happened at school—a classmate may have made fun of them in front of everyone or a teacher may have scolded them a little too harshly.

Adults, on the other hand, often complain of rheumatic pains in the joints of their hands or feet which baffle the doctors or turn out to be rheumatoid arthritis. On the cellular level the body is still carrying the trauma of an intense family quarrel that happened over two years before, or grieving the death of a beloved grandmother, grandfather, or other relation.

I unblock my stagnant energy and allow it to circulate freely.
I leave behind the traumatic visions of my past.
In interior peace, I reorient myself toward the light.

SKIN ZONES OF STAR OF BETHLEHEM

A   Frontal zone: area beginning in the middle of the forehead, extending downward to the intersection of the eyebrows and horizontally

1½ finger widths to the left and right of the midline.
Massage: *light*.

B   Left eye zone: area covering the left eye, beginning at the lower edge of the eyebrow and ending at the lower edge of the eye socket, extending horizontally from the inner margin of the iris to the outer tip of the eyebrow.
Massage: *light*.

C   Neck zone: area ⅜ inch in diameter located ¾ inch above the innermost part of the clavicle on the front of the neck.
Massage: *strong*.

D   Bilateral shoulder zone: area 1 inch in diameter located at the level of the scapulohumeral articulation on the front of both shoulders.
Massage: *light*.

E   Anterior thoracic zone: 1-inch-high rectangular area on the chest extending from above the horizontal line passing through the middle of the sternum and intersecting with the median clavicular line.
Massage: *light*.

F   Left inner arm zone: area ⅜ inch in diameter on the front of the left arm located 2 finger widths above the fold of the elbow and ¾ inch to the inside of the axial line.
Massage: *light*.

G   Bilateral wrist zone: oval area located on the inner fold of the wrist on both the left and right arms.
Massage: *light*.

H   Left thigh zone: area 1 inch in diameter located 4 finger widths above the upper edge of the kneecap on the front of the left thigh.
Massage: *light*.

I   Right foot zone: area ⅜ inch in diameter located on the top of the right foot ⅜ inch to the inside of the axial line of the foot and 2 finger widths below the fold of the ankle.
Massage: *light*.

J Right foot zone: area covering the top of the right foot from the tip of the little toe to the fold of the ankle.
Massage: *light.*

K Right posterior leg zone: area 1 inch in diameter just above the end of the Achilles tendon on the back of the lower right leg.
Massage: *light.*

L Bilateral arm zone: rectangular area located to the inside of the median line of the arm, beginning at the bend of the elbow and extending halfway up the upper arm on both sides of the body.
Massage: *light.*

M Dorsal zone: rectangular area located on the median vertebral line, extending from the first to the eighth lumbar vertebra.
Massage: *light.*

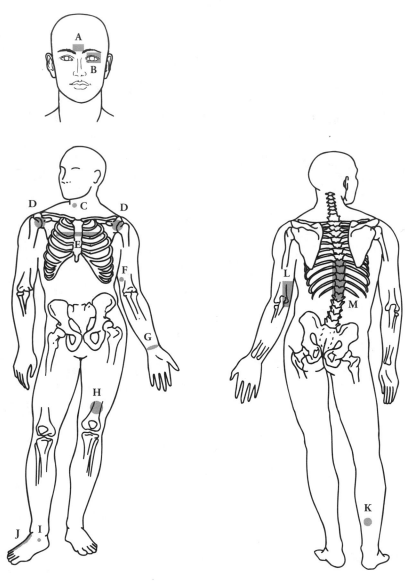

STAR OF BETHLEHEM

30
Sweet Chestnut
Castanea sativa Miller

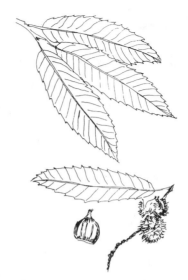

Family: Fagaceae

Habitat: Spontaneous and widespread in the eastern Mediterranean and cultivated elsewhere in Europe. Prefers loose, deep, siliceous soils and grows on hills and mountains up to 3,200 feet. Found in chestnut copses, it is nonetheless often associated with beech, spruce, pine, and oak.

Description: A long-lived tree that may reach over 500 years of age. Majestic in appearance, with a massive trunk and a rounded, spreading crown, it can be 112 feet high with a diameter of 26 feet. The trunk is straight and the bark is smooth, shiny, and dark red on the young limbs, turning a grayish olive green with time. The round, white lenticels on the younger branches are characteristic. After about 20 years the bark begins to furrow and crack, giving rise to a thick rhytidome mixed with dead tissue that forms large, long, dark gray ropes that may grow in a lefthand or righthand spiral. The deciduous leaves are up to 8 inches long and spiraled due to the twisting of their stems. Elliptical to lanceolate with toothed, crenated edges, they are an intense shining green on the right side and a lighter green on the underside; when young they are slightly pubescent. There are two types of catkins, which differ from each other in structure, order of appearance, and development of the inflorescence and flower: male and mixed. The male inflorescences, formed at the base of the branch, are composed of male flowers arranged in cymes or axillary glomerules of 7 flowers each; to every catkin there are about 40 cymes. The mixed inflorescences are found at the tip of the branch; the axillary cymes of the base are composed of 3 female flowers, while those at the summit consist of 2 male flowers. There are generally between 1 and 4 female cymes in each inflorescence. At first the flower presents itself as bisexual, with both male and female organs. The ovary, however, does not develop in the male catkins, while in the mixed catkins the stamens of the basal female flowers do not reach maturity. The 8 to 12 stamens of the male flower are extremely polliniferous and have a very penetrant odor. The female flowers are protected by scales that after fertilization form the husk. The ovary is inferior with 6 to 8 loculi and 4 to 9 styles that are rigid and hairy at the base. Sweet chestnut flowers from June through July.

Qualities:

- Total integration
- Rebirth
- Certainty of success in difficult situations
- Enlivened faith and self-confidence
- Belief
- Illumination on the path
- Emergence from utter despair
- Renewed joy in living
- Perception of one's bond with the Divine
- Inner clarity

Indicated for: those who feel deprived of every hope and live in the most extreme anguish, desperate because they feel that there is no way out. Perpetually tormented by life and their inner experiences, they view the world as a place of unrelieved suffering where nothing ever goes right, and ask no more than to pass to a better existence. Since they are shrouded in the deepest darkness and can glimpse not even the thinnest ray of light by which to orient themselves, they feel abandoned by God and everyone else. How many people, faced with misfortune, natural catastrophes, or a loved one's long and terminal illness, invoke an end to life and lose their faith!

The limit to what a human being can bear is reached, and it is necessary to cross the threshold of the impossible to be reborn, fulfill an evolution of the spirit, and transcend the illusion of reality. From a process that takes place in the shadows, in an extreme and abandoned solitude, the self is reborn and finds once again its essential, indispensible place in the world.

Children who need Sweet Chestnut are sad, apathetic, and isolated. Teased and turned away by their companions, they never smile and can react violently to taunts out of sheer desperation.

❦❦❦

I glimpse a faint light toward which I can steer.
I am reborn into a new life.
I believe in myself, in others, and in the Divine Principle.

❦❦❦

SKIN ZONES OF SWEET CHESTNUT

A Head zone: rectangular area on the top of the head, beginning at the hairline and ending 3 finger widths behind it, extending 1½ inches to the left and right of the midline.
Massage: *light.*

B Left eye zone: area covering the inside corner of the left eye, extending from the eyebrow to the lower edge of the eye socket and horizontally from the inner edge of the eye socket to the vertical line passing through the inner third of the eyebrow.
Massage: *light.*

C Right parietal zone: 2-inch-wide rectangular area extending from the horizontal line passing through the tip of the right ear downward to the point where the earlobe connects with the jaw.
Massage: *light.*

D Left retromandibular zone: small area between the temporomandibular joint and the mastoid on the left side of the neck.
Massage: *light.*

E Right shoulder zone: area 1 inch in diameter located 1 finger width
to the inside of the anterior axillary line on the front of the right
shoulder, 2 finger widths below the acromion.
Massage: *strong.*

F Left elbow zone: area ⅜ inch in diameter located 1 finger width
above the inner fold of the elbow on the lateral line of the left
arm.
Massage: *light.*

G Left side zone: rectangular area extending from the horizontal
line passing through the navel upward to the lower edge of the rib
cage. Its medial margin aligns vertically with the left nipple, its
lateral margin with the front axial fold.
Massage: *light.*

H Left forearm zone: rectangular area on the inner side of the lower
third of the left forearm.
Massage: *light.*

I Bilateral femoral zone: area 1 inch in diameter located at the top
of the femur on the lateral line of both sides of the body.
Massage: *light.*

J Medial left thigh zone: rectangular area on the inside of the left
thigh, beginning 1 finger width below the fold of the buttock
and ending 5 finger widths above the kneecap. The front border
is located 1 finger width to the inside of the kneecap and the zone
extends inward 3 finger widths.
Massage: *light.*

K Anterior left thigh zone: area 1 inch in diameter located 4 finger
widths from the upper edge of the left kneecap on the front of the
thigh.
Massage: *light.*

L Right knee zone: area 1 inch in diameter just above the right kneecap.
Massage: *light.*

M Lower left leg zone: area ⅜ inch in diameter located on the lower left leg 1 finger width in front of the lateral line and 4 inches above the fold of the ankle.
Massage: *light.*

N Right foot zone: rectangular area that covers the top of the right foot from the fold of the ankle down to the tip of the fourth and the outer half of the third toe.
Massage: *light.*

O Right buttock zone: area 1 inch in diameter located in the center of the right buttock.
Massage: *light.*

P Bilateral buttock zone: area covering the inner surface of both buttocks.
Massage: *light.*

Q Posterior right thigh zone: area ¼ inch in diameter located 4 inches below the superior anterior iliac spine on the lateral line of the body on the back of the right thigh.
Massage: *light.*

R Posterior left leg zone: area ⅜ inch in diameter about 4 inches below the fold of the knee and ⅜ inch behind the internal lateral line on the back of the left leg.
Massage: *light.*

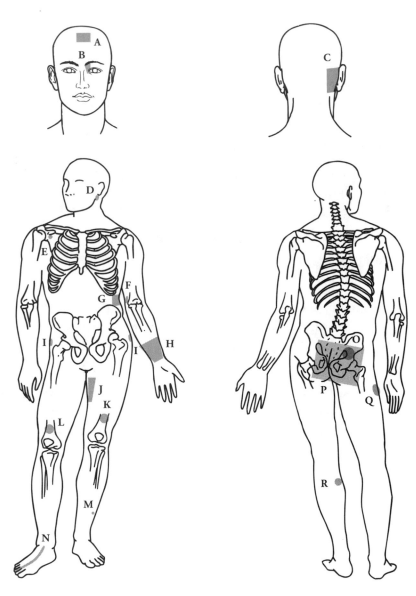

SWEET CHESTNUT

31
Vervain
Verbena officinalis

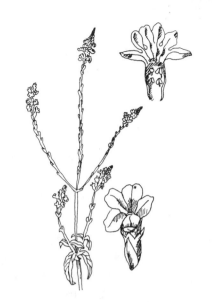

Family: Verbenaceae

Habitat: Present in its woodland form throughout most of Europe except in the extreme north and introduced in North America, vervain grows in uncultivated soils, among underbrush and shrubbery, in rubble, and along the edges of paths in plains and on hills and mountains up to 4,800 feet.

Description: A perennial, herbaceous, upright, downy plant up to 32 inches in height. The stalk is thin, viscous, and squarish, with protruding angles, and rough at the edges. The lower leaves are opposite, narrow, more or less deeply lobed, hirsute, and ¾ to 3 inches long. The 3- to 5-inch-long inflorescences are formed on leafless spikes borne on the branches; the flowers are 1½ inches in diameter, composed of a tubular corolla of 5 unequal petals and 4 enclosed stamens and a pubescent calyx with 5 teeth. Vervain flourishes from June to October.

Qualities:

- ≫ Ability to listen
- ≫ Flexibility
- ≫ Ability to allow others personal space
- ≫ Capacity to be oneself
- ≫ Respect for the feelings and opinions of others

- ⁊ Dissolution of fanaticism
- ⁊ Comprehension
- ⁊ Harmony between personal will and the world
- ⁊ Acceptance of life's rhythms
- ⁊ Engagement of energy with love

Indicated for: those who are continually driven by will and the desire to convince others that their ways of thinking and operating are the best ones, and everyone should follow suit. They can mesmerize the crowd, and are inexhaustible preachers and indefatigable organizers, often becoming missionaries. Impulsive, idealistic fighters, they cannot bear injustice and exaggerate to the point of fanaticism.

Since they are always in a state of inner and outer tension, they use up an enormous amount of energy and willpower. If they hit an obstacle that limits a given situation, they will suddenly lose energy and enthusiasm completely, becoming apathetic. Their friends no longer know them, saying, "But you used to be so stubborn and willful! Now here you are apathetic and listless."

Vervain children are very sure of themselves in the midst of their peers, and try to involve everyone in their games, which must be played exactly their way. Involved in a million things at once, they are lovers of justice and will quarrel with a companion who subjects another child to abuse. You can hear them coming by the noise they make walking, almost as if they were marching. They fight for their rights, which they defend fiercely, even when confronting a teacher. Vervain is also useful for children who are restless and overactive in the evening and who have trouble falling asleep because of mental tension.

I express my will out of a desire to respect others.
I adapt myself in harmony to the world.
My mental rigidity melts in the rhythmic flow of existence.

Skin Zones of Vervain

A   Right cheek zone: area on the right cheek whose upper margin aligns horizontally with the bottom of the nose and whose lower margin aligns horizontally with the right corner of the mouth. The outside margin aligns vertically with the outer end of the right eyebrow, while the inside border curves from the nose to the corner of the mouth.
Massage: *light*.

B   Bilateral neck zone: area on both sides of the neck, beginning 2 finger widths below the ear, aligned vertically with the back of the ear, and extending downward to the base of the neck and along the base of the neck to the collarbone. The front edge is formed by the ridge of the sternocleidomastoid muscle.
Massage: *light*.

C   Right thoracic zone: area below the right collarbone extending to the front of the fold of the armpit and downward, continuing along the costal arch and ending on a horizontal line 3 finger widths beneath the sternum.
Massage: *light*.

D   Right thoracic zone: area ⅜ inch in diameter near the median clavicular line, 4 finger widths above the edge of the rib cage on the right side of the chest.
Massage: *light*.

E   Bilateral femoral zone: area 1 inch in diameter located on the lateral line of the body at the level of the top of the femur on both the left and right legs.
Massage: *light*.

F   Right pubic-inguinal zone: small rectangular area beginning at the anterior median line and extending to cover the right side of the pubic mound and part of the groin.
Massage: *light*.

G   Right knee zone: area 1 inch in diameter located just above the right kneecap.
Massage: *light.*

H   Left knee zone: area ⅜ inch in diameter located ¾ inch below the left kneecap and ⅜ inch to the outside of the axial line of the leg.
Massage: *strong.*

I   Left shoulder zone: rectangular area extending from the horizontal median line of the scapula to the paravertebral and clavicular lines of the body, on the back of the left shoulder blade.
Massage: *light.*

J   Right dorsal zone: rectangular area beginning at the level of the second thoracic vertebra and ending at the level of the fifth thoracic vertebra, aligning vertically with the back axial fold and extending 3 finger widths toward midline on the right side of the back.
Massage: *light.*

K   Left dorsal zone: area ⅜ inch in diameter located 2 finger widths to the outside of the median clavicular line and horizontally aligned with the middle of the upper arm, on the left side of the back.
Massage: *strong.*

L   Left dorsal zone: area ⅜ inch in diameter located on the median clavicular line 4 finger widths below the scapula on the left side of the back.
Massage: *strong.*

M   Bilateral arm zone: rectangular area located to the inside of the median line, beginning at the bend of the elbow and continuing halfway up the upper arm on both the left and the right arms.
Massage: *light.*

N   Right palm zone: area ⅜ inch in diameter located on the hypothenar eminence 1 finger width below the fold of the wrist, on the axial line of the fourth finger of the right hand.
Massage: *light.*

O Right lower leg zone: area 1 inch in diameter just above the Achilles tendon on the back of the lower right leg.
Massage: *light.*

P Right foot zone: area beginning at the upper edge of the right ankle bone and ending at the lower edge of the right foot. The back border is formed by the Achilles tendon; the front border hugs the back of the outer ankle bone and runs in a slope toward the front.
Massage: *light.*

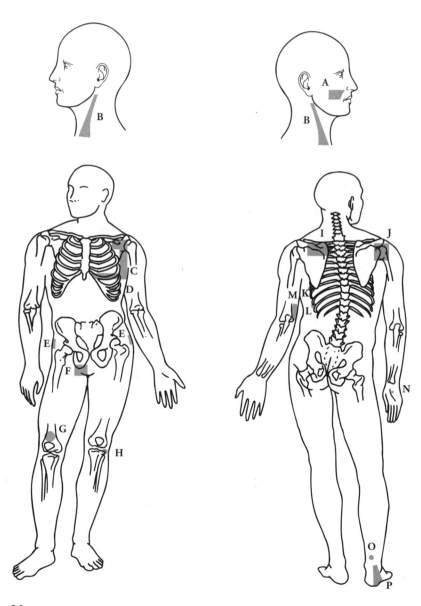

VERVAIN

32
Vine
Vitis vinifera (Grape vine)

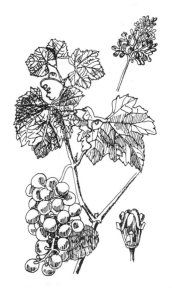

Family: Vitaceae

Habitat: Native to the southwest coasts of the Caspian Sea and widespread throughout Europe in the wake of its cultivation, becoming a symbol of European and especially Mediterranean civilization. It is now cultivated throughout the world in countries with temperate climates.

Description: A robust, woody, climbing vine that may reach 10 feet in height, although it is generally pruned back to a low shrub on an annual basis. The twisting trunk has rough bark that peels off in longitudinal strips and bears long, flexible shoots. The leaves are lobed, denticulate, heart-shaped, and deciduous; the vine shoots are supported by branching tendrils. The tiny, greenish flowers are unisexual and arranged in panicles. The hermaphroditic flower is pedunculate and furnished with a receptacle containing a gamosepalous calyx in the shape of a chalice marked by 5 miniscule notches and a 5-petaled corolla. This corolla falls off at maturity, revealing 5 stamens, each furnished with an anther with 2 pollinatory sacks supported by a filament. The pistil is solitary, formed by an ovary of 2 to 3 carpels, with 2 ovules per carpel. The dioecious flowers are characteristic of the American species. In the male flowers the gynaeceum is trophic and the stamens vigorous; in the female flowers the stamens produce sterile pollen. In Mediterranean climates vine flowers from March through April.

Qualities:

- Understanding
- Service to one's fellow human beings
- Wisdom in the guidance of others
- Gentleness and kindness
- Natural authority
- Service to the Higher Power
- Slaking of the thirst for power
- Respect

Indicated for: those who understand their own capacities, strengths, and affective will and are conscious of their own virtues. Habitually successful, they feel themselves to be winners and suffer from overinflated egos. Readily assuming the role of guide, they sometimes lose the thread of collaboration and become authoritarian and despotic, demanding complete and total obedience and walking all over anyone who interferes with their projects. They become tyrannical dictators, inspiring hatred, resentment, and rancor in their fellows. When these people achieve posts of prestige, they turn hard and rigid and make all their own laws, never stooping to compromise. Vine is the remedy of choice for anyone who believes that "the end justifies the means."

Even as very young children Vine people are leaders and lawmakers, tyrannical with their schoolmates to the point of becoming violent when their orders are not obeyed. They frequently rebel against their teachers and parents, especially if they are ordered to do something that puts them in a subordinate position.

In humility and understanding
I place myself at the service of others.
I serve the spirit within me.
I respect others and am developing a comprehension of their needs.

Skin Zones of Vine

A   Left parietal zone: area on the left side of the head, beginning 1½ finger widths to the side of midline and ending 3 finger widths above the top of the left ear. The back edge aligns with the tip of the ear and extends forward 3 finger widths.
Massage: *light.*

B   Right arm zone: area on the upper right arm beginning at the level of the fold of the armpit and ending 6 finger widths above the elbow. The front margin runs along the outside edge of the biceps; the back margin lies 3 finger widths to the right of the back axial fold.
Massage: *light.*

C   Right hand zone: area ⅜ inch in diameter located on the back of the right hand on the line of the fourth interdigital space, 1 inch from the bend of the wrist.
Massage: *strong.*

D   Bilateral shoulder zone: area 1 inch in diameter located on the posterior axial line on the back of both shoulders.
Massage: *light.*

E   Left dorsal zone: area ⅜ inch in diameter located on the median clavicular line 4 finger widths below the scapula on the left side of the back.
Massage: *strong.*

F   Lumbosacral zone: extends for about 1½ inches to the left and right of the line of the lower vertebrae.
Massage: *light.*

G   Right palm zone: area ⅜ inch in diameter located on the hypothenar eminence 1 finger width below the fold of the wrist on the axial line of the fourth finger of the right hand.
Massage: *light.*

H   Right palm zone: area covering the little finger and half of the ring finger of the right hand, extending down the palm to the

fold of the wrist.
Massage: *light.*

I   Lower right leg zone: area 1 inch in diameter just above the Achilles tendon on the back of the lower right leg.
Massage: *light.*

J   Left hand zone: area ⅜ inch in diameter located on the back of the left hand on the line of the fourth interdigital space, halfway between that space and the bend of the wrist.
Massage: *strong.*

K   Left palm zone: area ⅜ inch in diameter located at the level of the thenar eminence on the line of the first interdigital space of the left palm.
Massage: *light.*

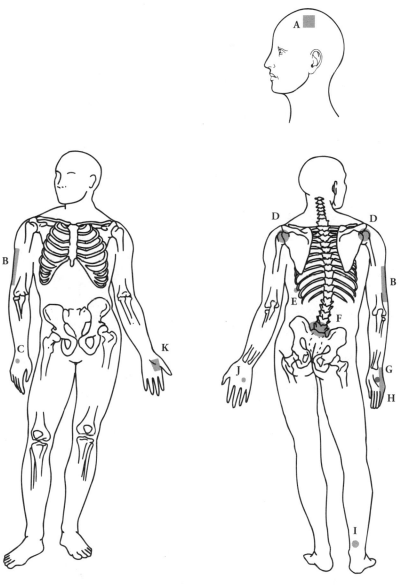

VINE

33
Walnut
Juglans regia

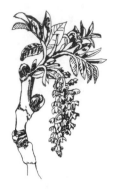

Family: Juglandaceae

Habitat: Originating in the temperate regions of central and western Asia and becoming widespread through cultivation in most of Europe since antiquity, walnut was introduced in England by the Romans. Since the massive exodus of European peasants from the countryside to the cities, however, older generations of walnut have been cut down without being replanted, and the tree is becoming ever rarer. Walnut thrives in deep and well-watered soils. A light-loving tree, it is not very sociable and does not tolerate other trees near it, so it is seldom found in forests.

Description: A tree that may reach 80 feet in height and 30 years in age, having a regular, rounded crown. The opaque silvery white bark remains smooth for a long time and then begins to crack into longitudinal furrows. The leaves are alternate, pinnate, compound, deciduous, and up to 16 inches long, formed by 5 to 9 ovate leaflets with pointed tips borne on a communal stem. The flowers are monoecious. The male flowers are borne on 3- to 3½-inch-long dark green catkins with numerous yellow stamens, situated at the axil of the preceding year's branchlets, while the female flowers are borne in groups of 2 to 5, located at the tips of this year's twigs.

Qualities:

- Freedom from external influences
- Shattering of the chains that bind one
- Self-confidence and ease
- Change and transformation
- Fulfillment
- Security
- Clarity regarding change undertaken

Indicated for: people who are hypersensitive and easily influenced, incapable of breaking the bonds that imprison their wills and lull to sleep any desire for change, growth, and renewal. Whenever they must make a major decision in life, they feel bound hand and foot to the memories, influences, and biases of the past. They hesitate to flout accepted convention and live forever according to their parents' expectations, because they are still influenced by their opinions and judgements. Such chronological adults are actually still children, very much in need of guidance.

Walnut is useful to persons in the process of giving birth to a new life, who have chosen to make the decisive move but who are not completely free, since they perceive the ties that bind them to the past. They want to start from scratch, but their feet are still planted on the shore of the old world. It is hard for them to accede to the new, to throw themselves freely toward physical or psychic renewal; they are unable to muster the force, vitality, and courage to do so.

As children they are afraid to go on to middle school or high school. Since they are also afraid to try new games with their friends, they always want to play the same old boring games over and over. They hate to change home, school, friends, or teachers.

I dissolve my ties with the past and turn toward the new.
I listen to the inner voice of renewal.
I find the strength and the will to be born anew.

Skin Zones of Walnut

A   Right eye zone: area located on the inside corner of the right eye, extending from the eyebrow to the lower rim of the eye socket and from the inside edge of the iris to the midpoint between the eyebrows.
Massage: *light*.

B   Nose zone: area ⅜ inch in diameter located on the median line at the base of the nose on the left side of the face.
Massage: *light*.

C   Left elbow zone: area ⅜ inch in diameter 1 finger width above the inner fold of the elbow on the lateral median line of the left arm.
Massage: *light*.

D   Bilateral femoral zone: area 1 inch in diameter located on the lateral line of the body at the level of the top of the femur on both the left and right hip.
Massage: *light*.

E   Left thigh zone: area 1 inch in diameter located on the front of the left thigh 4 finger widths above the upper edge of the kneecap.
Massage: *light*.

F   Left knee zone: area ⅜ inch in diameter located just above the upper edge of the left kneecap and 2 finger widths to the outside of the axial line.
Massage: *strong*.

G   Left knee zone: medium-sized rectangular area located on the front of the left knee.
Massage: *light*.

H   Bilateral knee zone: area 1 inch in diameter located on the median line of both the left and right knees.
Massage: *light*.

I Right lower thigh zone: area 1 inch in diameter located above the kneecap on the lower front part of the right thigh.
Massage: *light.*

J Right lower leg zone: area ⅜ inch in diameter located on the lower right leg 3 inches above the inner ankle bone and ¾ inch in front of the lateral line.
Massage: *light.*

K · Posterior right leg zone: area 1 inch in diameter located just above the Achilles tendon on the back of the lower right leg.
Massage: *light.*

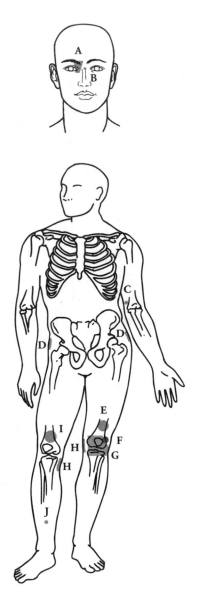
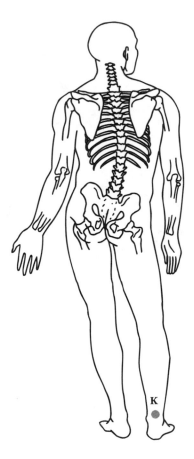

WALNUT

34
Water Violet
Hottonia palustris

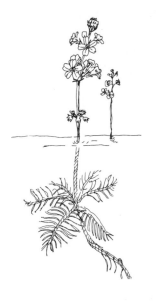

Family: Primulaceae

Habitat: Spontaneous throughout a vast region extending from western Siberia to all of northern and central Europe, water violet thrives in stagnant water in marshes and ditches.

Description: Perennial, acquatic, floating, rhyzomatic plant up to 2 feet high. The leaves are submerged, pinnate, and separated into entire, linear, fringed, and capillariform segments forming a rosette around the flower-bearing stem, which grows upward out of the water. The large flowers borne on this stalk form long, hairy, glandular racemes, structurally well adapted to impollination by insects, confirming the plant's descent from ancient terrestrial forebears. The dimorphous flowers vary in color from white to pink and lavender and secrete nectar. The calyx is divided into 5 linear laciniae; the corolla is formed of 5 emarginate, deep, irregular lobes, with a thickened throat and grooved petals. The 5 stamens are enclosed and are as long as the calyx. The ovary is spherical and the style is persistent in the fruit. Water violet flowers from May through July.

Qualities:

>≈ Communication
>≈ Humility

- Integration with others
- Sympathy
- Serenity
- Service
- Amiability
- Dissolution of superiority complex
- Inner balance
- Openness
- Capacity to share with joy

Indicated for: people who feel they live in a castle and believe themselves perfectly able to live in isolation, confident in their self-sufficiency. They don't want to interfere in things, prefer solitude, and choose to share nothing—not even their emotions—with others. They are so excessively reserved as to become rigid and haughty and appear very aristocratic, inaccessible to the rest of us mortals. They spend a great deal of energy maintaining this modus vivendi, or they block it in certain areas of the body, often creating aches and pains and rigidity of the joints.

People in need of this remedy exist in a lethargic state, tucked into their turtle shells, despising and avoiding the world and humanity.

As children they appear mature for their age, already speaking like adults and aloof from the play of their peers. They are too proud to ask for help and are rigid in their movements and expressions. Should a teacher reach out in a gesture of sympathy or affection, the Water Violet child is sure to withdraw.

I share my world with others.
I open myself to love and give love to others.
I nourish in myself a spirit of communion with the cosmos.

Skin Zones of Water Violet

A   Frontal zone: rectangular area in the middle of the forehead beginning at the hairline, ending halfway between the hairline and the midpoint of the eyebrows, and extending 1½ finger widths to the left and right of the midline.
Massage: *light.*

B   Right temple zone: 1-inch-wide rectangular area located on the surface of the right temple, extending from the outer tip of the right eyebrow down to where the horizontal line passing through the lower rim of the eye socket meets the hairline in front of the ear.
Massage: *light.*

C   Posterior neck zone: rectangular area on the back of the neck extending from the sixth cervical vertebra to the occipital base, with a width of almost 2½ inches.
Massage: *light.*

D   Anterior neck zone: area located on the front of the neck, extending vertically from the middle of the Adam's apple to the upper rim of the sternum and bordered on both sides by the sternocleidomastoid muscles.
Massage: *light.*

E   Epigastric zone: oval area with its center halfway between the navel and the xiphoid process.
Massage: *light.*

F   Bilateral wrist zone: oval area located on the inner fold of the wrist of both the left and right arms.
Massage: *light.*

G   Left palm zone: area ⅜ inch in diameter located on the hypothenar eminence 1 finger width below the inner fold of the wrist on the fourth interdigital line of the left palm.
Massage: *light.*

H   Left foot zone: area extending from the fold of the left ankle and running down the back of the left foot to the tip of the little toe.
Massage: *light.*

I   Right dorsal zone: area ⅜ inch in diameter located on the right side of the back, 4 finger widths below the scapula and 2 finger widths from the median line.
Massage: *strong.*

J   Lumbosacral zone: extends for about 1½ inches to the left and right of the lower line of the spinal vertebrae.
Massage: *light.*

K   Right buttock zone: narrow rectangular area extending from the upper third of the right buttock to its fold.
Massage: *light.*

L   Lower left leg zone: area ⅜ inch in diameter located on the back of the lower left leg, ¾ inch below the midpoint of the calf and 1 finger width to the outside of the posterior axial line.
Massage: *light.*

M   Left ankle zone: area encircling the lower part of the left leg, beginning at the upper edge of the ankle bone and extending 4 finger widths upward around the leg.
Massage: *light.*

N   Posterior right leg zone: area 1 inch in diameter just above the Achilles tendon on the back of the right lower leg.
Massage: *light.*

O   Left hand zone: area ⅜ inch in diameter located on the back of the left hand on the line of the fourth interdigital space, midway between that space and the bend of the wrist.
Massage: *strong.*

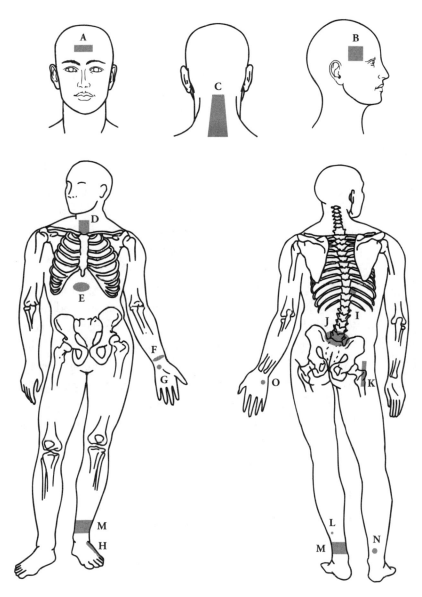

WATER VIOLET

35
White Chestnut
Aesculus hippocastanum (Horsechestnut)

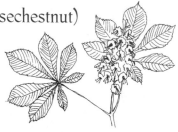

Family: Hippocastanaceae

Habitat: Originally native to southeastern Europe in the Caucasus and the Balkans, introduced in western and northern Europe in the sixteenth century, and widely planted throughout North America, it now grows wild in the northeastern United States.

Description: A large, elegant, short-lived tree up to 75 feet in height with a dense, regular, rounded crown. The bark is a dark reddish or grayish color and flakes off in big scaly plates. The palmate, compound leaves are opposite and carried on a long, rough stalk. They form a fan shape as 7 to 9 wedge-shaped, toothed, unequal leaflets radiating from a common point. The buds are large and very sticky. The large bisexual flowers have bilateral symmetry and are white, spotted red and yellow at the base, and borne in conical, upright, branched clusters. The calyx has 4 unequal teeth; the corolla has 4 unequal and undulate petals; there are 7 to 9 stamens and 1 protruding style; and the ovary is divided into 3 lobes. The familiar shiny brown nuts are found within the three-part green husk.

    Caution: These nuts are poisonous and must not be eaten, as they contain a dangerous glycoside.

Qualities:

    ➤ Peace and inner tranquility
    ➤ Mental freedom

- Diminution of obsessive thinking
- Dissolution of redundancy
- Interest in the present situation
- Appropriate focus in thinking
- Capacity to direct thought
- Mental clarity
- Inner quiet

Indicated for: persons who seem to have a kind of "thought machine" inside their heads and repeat themselves obsessively, always harping on the same subject. It seems that they never go forward in life, but are stuck at one point and just keep circling around it. After a while everything gets confused and agonizingly painful.

They come home after work and brood on what they could have done differently that day: "I should have said . . . What I could have done . . . I wish I had listened to that advice."

It seems they have no interest in the present situation but live in remembrance of the past, and the thoughts and ideas that guide them pile up so quickly that finally their brains feel like valleys of zigzagging echoes. The mental energy is all there, trapped by the skull, with no way out to expand toward new experiences.

As children their brains are constantly working, like little manufacturing plants that never shut down. They come to lack imagination, since they cannot manage to stop the flow of their thoughts. They become inconclusive and repetitive, and though apparently attentive when their friends talk they are actually absent, absorbed in their world of ideas. If called on to demonstrate what they know they tumble out of the clouds and ask someone to repeat the question.

I calm the storm of my thoughts.
I rekindle the light of clarity and calm.
I work toward a state of inner quiet.

SKIN ZONES OF WHITE CHESTNUT

A   Left parietal zone: area on the left side of the head whose lower border aligns with the tip of the ear, with the zone extending upward for 3 finger widths. The front border lies 3 finger widths behind the ear, with the zone extending backward for 3 finger widths. Massage: *light*.

B   Thoracic zone: area ⅜ inch in diameter located on the right parasternal in the fourth intercostal space on the front of the chest. Massage: *light*.

C   Right thoracic zone: area ⅜ inch in diameter located on the median axial line 3 finger widths below the fold of the armpit on the right side of the chest. Massage: *light*.

D   Left arm zone: area ⅜ inch in diameter located 2 finger widths from the fold of the elbow and ¾ inch from the axial line on the inner side of the left arm. Massage: *strong*.

E   Right leg zone: rectangular area on the back and side of the lower right leg extending from the horizontal line passing through the middle of the calf to 2 finger widths below the inner fold of the knee and from the posterior axial line to the ridge of the fibula. Massage: *light*.

F   Bilateral foot zone: area ⅜ inch in diameter located at the level of acupuncture point Sp2 on both feet. Massage: *light*.

G   Right shoulder zone: area ⅜ inch in diameter located ⅜ inch to the inside of the median clavicular line and ⅜ inch above the spine of the scapula on the back of the right shoulder. Massage: *strong*.

H   Bilateral shoulder zone: area 1 inch in diameter located on the posterior axial line on the back of both shoulders. Massage: *light*.

I Bilateral arm zone: rectangular area located to the inside of the median line, beginning at the bend of the elbow and extending halfway up the upper arm on both the left and right arms. Massage: *light*.

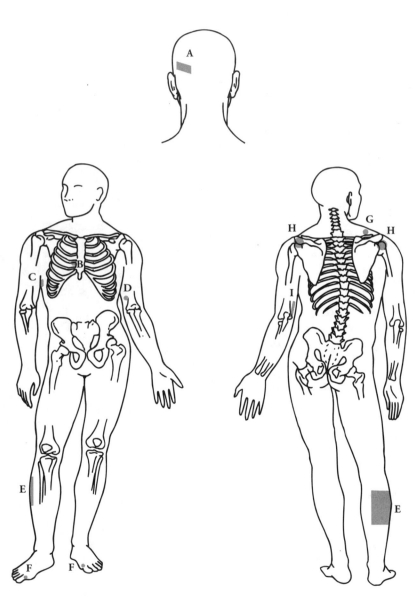

WHITE CHESTNUT

36
Wild Oat
Bromus ramosus

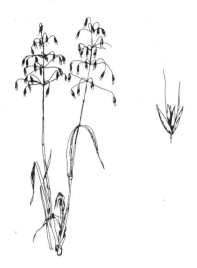

Family: Graminaceae

Habitat: Present in Europe on wooded slopes and in shady groves and copses.

Description: Herbaceous plant that can reach 5 feet in height. The green leaves form a sheath that wraps around the stalk. The inflorescence is limp and pendulous, formed by slender, spindle-shaped spikelets from ¾ to 1½ inches long with short, bristly awns. Wild oat flowers from June through August.

Qualities:

- Clarity of decision
- Determination
- Work resulting in tangible results
- Perseverance
- Vocation
- Lucidity
- Self-confidence
- Rootedness

Indicated for: those who are forever searching for something or someone else, or even themselves. They feel as though they are standing at a crossroads, trying to decide which way to take. None of their many ambitions is ever completely fulfilled; they stop halfway or three-quarters through, and that's it. Creative as well as ambitious, they have mutable characters and push themselves to carry out an enormous number of projects. They may change jobs twice a year and do not seem to quite understand their own attitudes or where they should settle. They can be cerebral wanderers.

In a kind of mental puberty, their brains continue to focus on what they need or might need. They seem to lack an interior guide, a beacon by which to orient themselves. They throw themselves into a thousand things and don't finish one.

Children who respond to Wild Oat are discontent and dissatisfied, since they never manage to bring their undertakings to any conclusion. They take hours to finish a theme or math problem, and will work hard on the rough work of carving a toy boat from a piece of wood only to set it down and abandon the project.

I walk the path I have taken to its end.
I mold my purpose in life with determination.
I create opportunities for self-fulfillment.

SKIN ZONES OF WILD OAT

A   Right thoracic zone: rectangular area beginning at the outer half of the right collarbone and ending at the third intercostal space. The outer margin aligns vertically with the axial line of the body; the inner margin lies 4 finger widths to the right of midline.
Massage: *light.*

B   Right arm zone: area ⅜ inch in diameter located between the ventral axial line and the external lateral line, 2 finger widths below the armpit on the upper right arm.
Massage: *strong.*

C   Lower right thoracic zone: area ⅜ inch in diameter located on the median axial line 3 finger widths below the fold of the armpit on the right side of the chest.
Massage: *light.*

D   Left elbow zone: area ⅜ inch in diameter located 1 finger width above the fold of the elbow on the lateral line on the inside of the upper left arm.
Massage: *light.*

E   Right hip zone: 2½-inch-wide rectangular area extending from the horizontal line passing through the navel down to the top of the femur on the right hip.
Massage: *light.*

F   Left thigh zone: area 1 inch in diameter located 4 finger widths above the upper edge of the kneecap on the front of the left thigh.
Massage: *light.*

G   Left knee zone: area ⅜ inch in diameter located just above the upper edge of the kneecap 2 finger widths to the outside of the axial line on the left leg.
Massage: *strong.*

H   Left lower leg zone: area ⅜ inch in diameter located 1 finger width in front of the lateral line and 4 inches above the fold of the ankle on the side of the lower left leg.
Massage: *light.*

I   Lumbosacral zone: rectangular area located at the level of the fifth lumbar vertebra, extending about 1½ inches to the left and right of the midline on the lower back.
Massage: *light.*

J   Posterior left thigh zone: area 1 inch in diameter located on the axial line halfway up the back of the left thigh.
Massage: *light.*

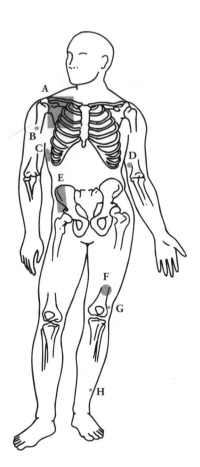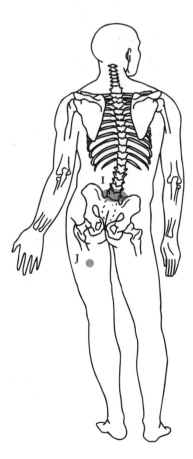

WILD OAT

37
Wild Rose
Rosa canina

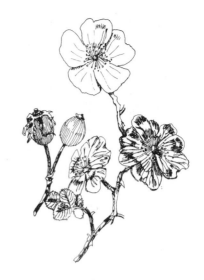

Family: Rosaceae

Habitat: Present in Europe in clearings, abandoned fields, hedges, woods, and undergrowth from sea level to 4,200 feet of altitude.

Description: A perennial shrub that may reach 12 feet in height. The stalk is green and armed with thorns, wide at the base, and very sharp at the tip; there are often also subterranean stems. The branches are erect in the lower part of the plant, drooping and armed with prickles toward the top. The leaves are pinnately compound and are composed of 5 or 7 elliptical, toothed, hairless leaflets with elongated stipules. The hermaphroditic flower varies between ¾ to 3¼ inches in diameter and is composed of a rather large, bottle-shaped calyx with 5 pink or white petals, triangular sepals, and numerous stamens. Wild rose flowers between June and July.

Qualities:

- Renewed interest in life
- Devotion
- Motivation
- Awareness
- Lively curiosity
- Vitality
- Ability to solve problems
- Strength to begin living again

- Dissolution of apathy and indifference
- Creativity
- Sensitivity to beauty

Indicated for: people who are inwardly resigned and give up before they've begun, who have trouble just waking up in the morning and take offense at a friendly "hello." Always tired, apathetic, and unmotivated, they believe in no ideals strongly enough to struggle toward them. Extremely withdrawn, they have trouble leaving the house and spend hours in front of the TV screen. Spiritually, they have abandoned all hope and initiative. Inwardly and outwardly, they are pervaded by a sense of resignation.

Life seems to deny these people any way out, and every situation turns into a dead end. At times their minds are a tumult of schemes and ideas, but these swiftly become illusions they must chase without any hope of capture. When queried about their apathy, they will answer, "I don't know," and they often sit in one place or lie stretched out on the couch for whole days at a time in a state of almost paralyzed indifference. Any joy of life has vanished like smoke. They have lost all inner motivation to act, and even their voices are low and monotonous.

Children in need of Wild Rose are equally apathetic—nothing really interests them; they go to school to warm their chairs; they are always sitting in front of the TV watching cartoons. Although their friends invite them out to play, they prefer to be alone, stretched out on the bed or the couch, doing nothing.

I rediscover the blessings of life, for which I must sometimes struggle.
I feel enthusiasm for the beauty of the earth, for humanity and life.
I acknowledge innumerable reasons for living
in harmony with the cosmos.

SKIN ZONES OF WILD ROSE

A Nose zone: area ⅜ inch in diameter located on the median line of

the nose at the level of the eyes.
Massage: *light.*

B   Right shoulder zone: area ⅜ inch in diameter located 1 finger width to the inside of the anterior axial line and 2 finger widths below the acromion on the front of the right shoulder.
Massage: *strong.*

C   Right forearm zone: rectangular area extending from the juncture of the ulnus and the humerus to the back of the elbow and from the bend of the elbow to the wrist of the right arm.
Massage: *light.*

D   Bilateral femoral zone: area 1 inch in diameter located at the level of the top of the femur on the lateral line of the body on both the left and right hip.
Massage: *light.*

E   Left buttock zone: rectangular area extending from the top of the femur to 1 finger width below the fold of the left buttock, whose front margin aligns vertically with the front axial fold. The zone extends backward 3 finger widths beyond the vertical line of the back axial fold and is elongated on the front of the left thigh in a small rectangle about 1½ inches high.
Massage: *light.*

F   Bilateral wrist zone: oval area located just above the inner fold of the wrist on both the left and right arms.
Massage: *light.*

G   Left thigh zone: area 1 inch in diameter located 4 finger widths above the upper edge of the kneecap on the front of the left thigh.
Massage: *light.*

H   Right leg zone: area ⅜ inch in diameter located 3 inches above the ankle bone and ¼ inch in front of the lateral line of the right leg.
Massage: *light.*

I   Right foot zone: area ⅜ inch in diameter located on the top of the right foot ⅜ inch to the inside of the median line and 2 finger

widths below the bend of the ankle.
Massage: *light.*

J   Left foot zone: area covering half of the big toe, half of the third toe, and all of the second toe on the left foot, running up the top of the foot to the bend of the ankle.
Massage: *light.*

K   Cervical zone: rectangular area covering the seventh cervical and first thoracic vertebrae, located at the level of the axial line.
Massage: *light.*

L   Lumbar zone: oval area covering the first lumbar vertebra.
Massage: *light.*

M   Bilateral arm zone: rectangular area located to the inside of the median line of both the left and right arms, beginning at the bend of the elbow and extending halfway up the upper arm.
Massage: *light.*

N   Right parietal zone: area extending from the vertical lines passing through the tip of the right ear and the acupuncture point GB20 and the horizontal lines passing through the inner third of the right eyebrow and the hairline.
Massage: *light.*

O   Right forearm zone: area on the dorsal side and inner third of the right forearm.
Massage: *light.*

P   Right posterior leg zone: area ⅜ inch in diameter located 1 inch below the inner fold of the knee and 1 finger width to the outside of the axial line on the back of the right leg.
Massage: *strong.*

Q   Left parietal zone: area on the left side of the top of the head, bordered in the front by the line passing through acupuncture point GB20 and in the back by the line passing through the inner third of the left eyebrow and the hairline.
Massage: light.

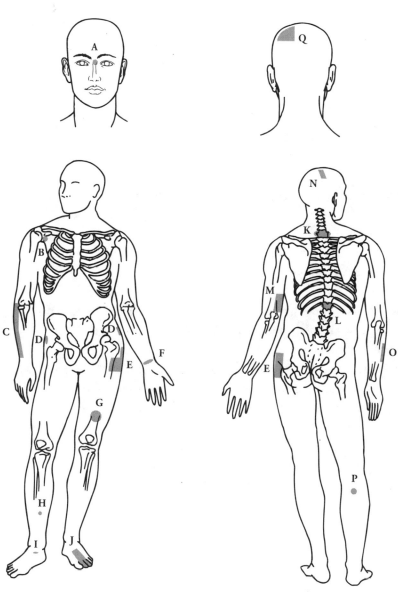

WILD ROSE

38
Willow
Salix vitellina

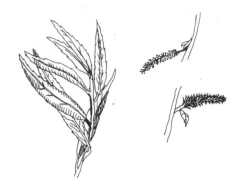

Family: Salicaceae

Habitat: Spontaneous along ditches and in valleys of central and southern Europe, North Africa, and Asia; present in North America from Nova Scotia and Ontario to Iowa, North Carolina, and Tennessee. It is not found in forests, but is widely cultivated for its willow rods, used in weaving baskets.

Description: A tree that may reach 80 feet in height, having a robust trunk, whose young branches are flexible and brilliant orange or yellow and are frequently cut back to the trunk when cultivated to encourage the luxuriant growth of pliable stems for use in basketry. The leaves are long and narrow, dark green, finely toothed, and have whitish, silky hair on both sides. The unisexual flowers, located on different plants, are carried on rigid, erect catkins with entire scales that form before the leaves. The perianth is composed of 1 or 2 nectar-bearing glands; there are 2 to 5 yellow stamens and 2 more or less entire stigmas. The male catkins are at first silvery gray and later turn yellow, while the female catkins are green and not very showy. Willow flowers between March and May.

Qualities:

- Relinquishment of rancor
- Self-purification and cleaning

- Freedom from guilt
- Self-responsibility
- Self-respect
- Dissolution of bitterness, resentment, and envy
- Mastery of one's own destiny
- Desire for transformation
- Relinquishment of the role of victim

Indicated for: people who feel persecuted by fate and treated unfairly, who perceive all that happens to them as coming from the outside world. They blame others for the failures of their lives and fall prey to bitterness, resentment, and rancor, becoming victims without understanding that the quality of their lives depends on them, the masters of their destinies. If instead they were luminous, joyful, and loving, their lives would also shine and bear better fruit.

But Willow people keep a black diary, in which they write down all their negative impressions and what they must remember to do to avenge the injustices done them. They project their delusions, angers, and sense of failure—of having lived always in reflected light without ever kindling their own—onto the outer world.

Children in need of this remedy constantly complain. They are innocent victims who never do anything wrong and always put the blame on their companions. Vindictive and disruptive, they may secretly kick a classmate under the desk or hide his schoolbag during exams. It is almost as if they wanted to replace fate, so harsh in its directives.

A new light dawns on my life to inspire me with hope and appreciation.
I dissolve the bitterness and envy I keep stored within me.
I guide my life with certainty and firmness.

Skin Zones of Willow

A Left neck zone: rectangular zone on the left side of the neck beginnning at the tip of the ear and extending to the base of the neck. The front margin follows the base of the ear and the zone extends 2 finger widths to the back.
Massage: *light*.

B Mouth zone: area beginning at the bottom of the nose and extending in a curve over the upper lip to the corners of the mouth, ending at the lower edge of the lower lip.
Massage: *light*.

C Left forearm zone: area ⅜ inch in diameter located 4 finger widths above the fold of the wrist and ⅜ inch in front of the internal lateral line of the left forearm.
Massage: *strong*.

D Bilateral wrist zone: oval area located on the inner fold of both the left and right wrists.
Massage: *light*.

E Right thigh zone: area 1 inch in diameter located above the right kneecap on the front of the thigh.
Massage: *light*.

F Left lower leg zone: area ⅜ inch in diameter located 1 finger width in front of the lateral line and 4 inches above the fold of the ankle on the lower left leg.
Massage: *light*.

G Right foot zone: area ⅜ inch in diameter located 2 finger widths below the fold of the ankle and ⅜ inch to the inside of the axial line on the top of the right foot.
Massage: *light*.

H Left arm zone: area beginning at the acromioclavicular joint of the shoulder and following the posterior axial line downward to end 3 finger widths below the tip of the elbow on the left arm.
Massage: *light*.

I Bilateral arm zone: rectangular area located to the inside of the median line of the arm, beginning at the elbow and extending halfway up the upper arm on both the left and right arms.
Massage: *light.*

J Right dorsal zone: area ⅜ inch in diameter located on the ridge of the clavicle, 2 finger widths above the edge of the rib cage.

K Right buttock zone: rectangular area high on the right buttock, beginning at the fifth lumbar vertebra and extending downward to the midpoint of the sacrum, extending horizontally from the paravertebral to the axial line.
Massage: *light.*

L Posterior right thigh zone: area ⅜ inch in diameter located ⅜ inch to the inside of the axial line and about 8 inches above the fold of the knee on the back of the right thigh.
Massage: *strong.*

M Posterior left thigh zone: area 1 inch in diameter located on the axial line halfway up the back of the left thigh.
Massage: *light.*

N Left popliteal zone: area covering the popliteal cave on the back of the left knee.
Massage: *light.*

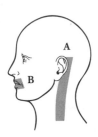

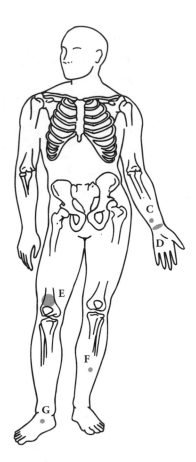

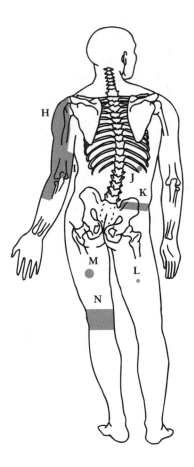

WILLOW

Resources

The original Bach Flower Remedies are still collected at the same sites used by Dr. Edward Bach and are prepared according to his method. These original flower essences can be purchased individually or as a complete set from the following suppliers:

North America

Ellon USA
644 Merrick Road
Lynbrook, NY 11563
Phone: (516) 593-2206
       (800) 423-2256
Fax: (516) 593-9668

England

Bach Flower Remedies Ltd.
Dr. Edward Bach Center
Mount Vernon
Sotwell, Wallingford
Oxfordshire OX10 0PZ

Healing Health Ltd.
P.O. Box 65
GB-Hereford HR2 OUW

Australia

The Pharmaceutical Plant
   Company
P.O. Box 68
Bayswater, Victoria 3153
Phone: 03-762 8577/8522

Martin & Pleasance Wholesale
   Pty Ltd.
P.O. Box 4
Collingwood, Victoria 3066
Phone: 419-9733

FURTHER READING

Bach, E. *Collected Writings.* Ed. J. Barnard. Hereford, England: Flower Remedy Programme, 1987.

Bach, E., and F. J. Wheeler. *The Bach Flower Remedies.* New Canaan, CT: Keats, 1979.

Barnard, J. *Patterns of Life Force.* Hereford, England: Flower Remedy Programme, 1987.

Barnard, J., and M. Barnard. *The Healing Herbs of Edward Bach: An Illustrated Guide to the Flower Remedies.* Bath, England: Ashgrove, 1988.

Chancellor, Philip. *The Handbook of the Bach Flower Remedies.* New Canaan, CT: Keats, 1980.

Cunningham, D. *Flower Remedies Handbook.* New York: Sterling, 1992.

Damian, Peter. *The Twelve Healers of the Zodiac: The Astrology Handbook of the Bach Flower Remedies.* York Beach, ME: Weiser, 1986.

Kaminski, P. *Flower Essence Repertory.* Nevada City, CA: Flower Essence Society, 1994.

Krämer, Dietmar. *New Bach Flower Therapies: Theory and Practice.* Rochester, VT: Healing Arts Press, 1995.

———. *New Bach Flower Body Maps.* Rochester, VT: Healing Arts Press, 1996.

Lo Rito, D. Iridotherapy. In *Iridology Review,* Vol. 1(3), 1992.

Mazzarella, Barbara. *Bach Flower Remedies for Children.* Rochester, VT: Healing Arts Press, 1997.

Scheffer, Mechthild. *Bach Flower Therapy: Theory and Practice.* Rochester, VT: Healing Arts Press, 1988.

———. *Mastering Bach Flower Therapies.* Rochester, VT: Healing Arts Press, 1996.

Vlamis, Gregory. *Bach Flower Remedies to the Rescue.* Rochester, VT: Healing Arts Press, 1990.

Weeks, Nora. *The Medical Discoveries of Edward Bach, Physician.* New Canaan, CT: Keats, 1979.

Healing Arts Press books may be ordered by calling 1-800-371-3174.

INDEX